KETO COMFORT FOODS

SAM
DILLARD
of HeyKetoMama.com
Author of *The "I Love My Air Fryer"
Keto Diet Recipe Book*

KETO
COMFORT
FOODS

100 KETO-FRIENDLY RECIPES FOR YOUR COMFORT-FOOD FAVORITES

3 1336 11061 6936

ADAMS MEDIA
NEW YORK LONDON TORONTO SYDNEY NEW DELHI

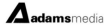

Adams Media
An Imprint of Simon & Schuster, Inc.
57 Littlefield Street
Avon, Massachusetts 02322

First Adams Media trade paperback edition December 2019

ADAMS MEDIA and colophon are trademarks of Simon & Schuster.

For information about special discounts for bulk purchases, please contact Simon & Schuster Special Sales at 1-866-506-1949 or business@simonandschuster.com.

The Simon & Schuster Speakers Bureau can bring authors to your live event. For more information or to book an event contact the Simon & Schuster Speakers Bureau at 1-866-248-3049 or visit our website at www.simonspeakers.com.

Interior design by Sylvia McArdle and Stephanie Hannus
Photographs by James Stefiuk

Manufactured in the United States of America

10 9 8 7 6 5 4 3 2 1

Library of Congress Cataloging-in-Publication Data
Names: Dillard, Sam, author.
Title: Keto comfort foods / Sam Dillard of HeyKetoMama.com, author of The "I love my air fryer" keto diet recipe book.
Description: Avon, Massachusetts: Adams Media, 2019.
Includes index.
Identifiers: LCCN 2019030582 | ISBN 9781507212202 (pb) | ISBN 9781507212219 (ebook)
Subjects: LCSH: Reducing diets--Recipes. | Ketogenic diet. | Comfort food. | LCGFT: Cookbooks.
Classification: LCC RM222.2 .D5753 2019 | DDC 641.5/635--dc23
LC record available at https://lccn.loc.gov/2019030582

ISBN 978-1-5072-1220-2
ISBN 978-1-5072-1221-9 (ebook)

Chapter 1 contains material adapted from the following title published by Adams Media, an Imprint of Simon & Schuster, Inc.: *The "I Love My Air Fryer" Keto Diet Recipe Book* by Sam Dillard, copyright © 2019, ISBN 978-1-5072-0992-9.

CONTENTS

CHAPTER 1

WHAT IS A KETO DIET? 12

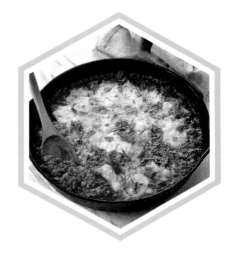

CHAPTER 2

KETO CASSEROLES 23

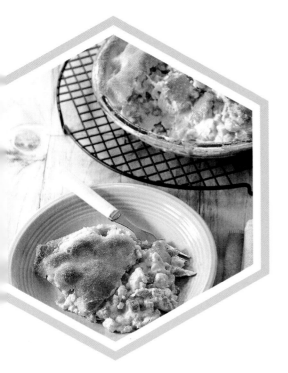

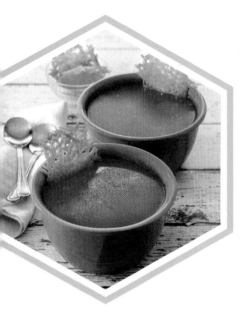

CHAPTER 4
KETO PIZZAS 63

CHAPTER 3
KETO SOUPS, STEWS, AND CHILIS 43

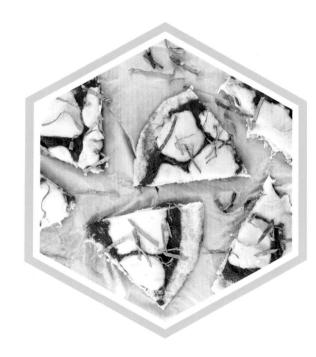

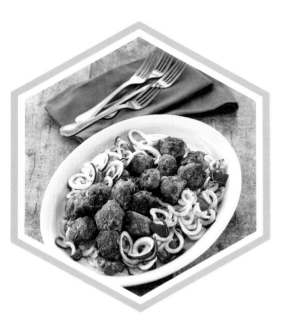

CHAPTER 6
KETO CLASSIC COMFORT DISHES 103

CHAPTER 5
KETO "RICE" AND "PASTAS" 83

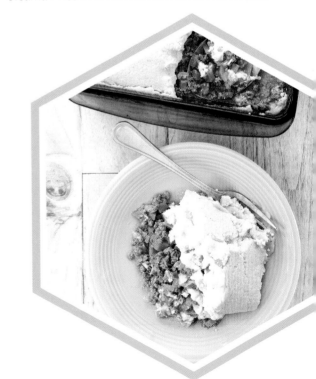

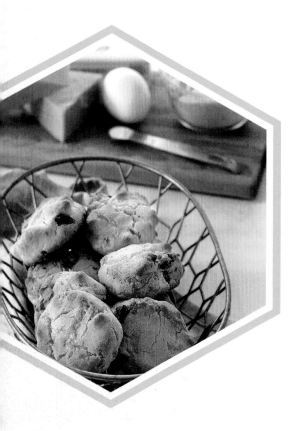

CHAPTER 7
KETO COMFORT SIDES 121

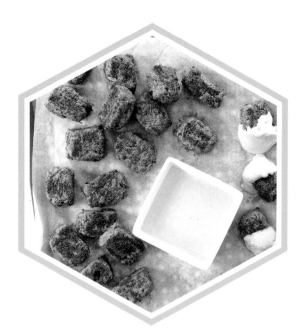

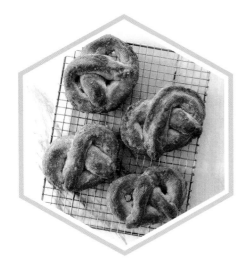

CHAPTER 8

KETO BAKED GOODS AND SWEETS 141

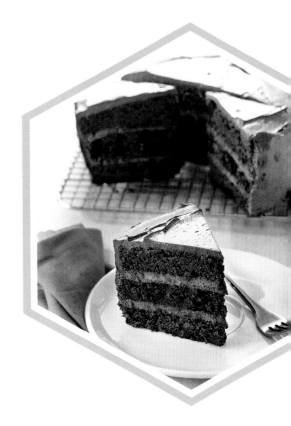

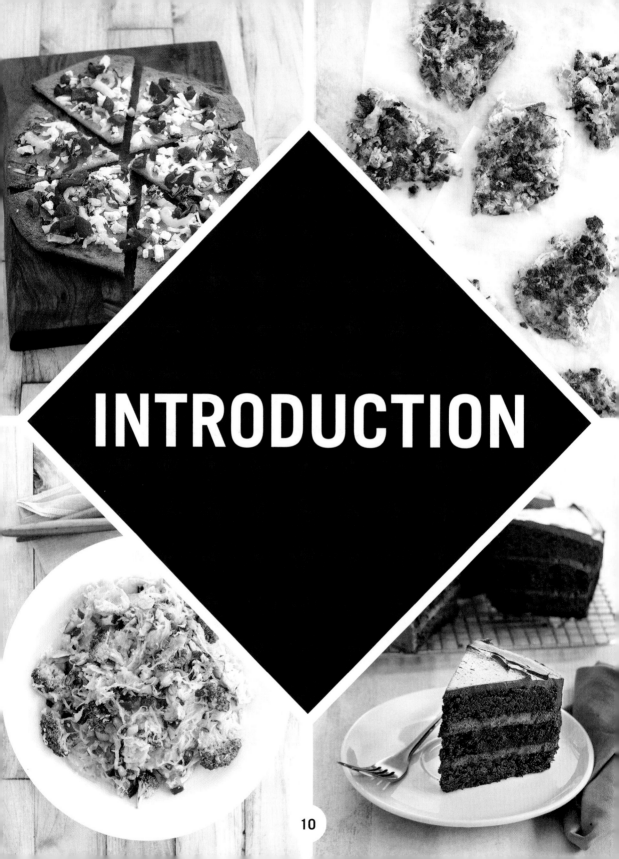

INTRODUCTION

Crustless Quiche Lorraine

Chicken Potpie Casserole

Cheeseburger Helper

Crispy Avocado Fry Nachos

Comfort foods make us feel good. Not only are they delicious; they also have a unique way of making us feel special. Unfortunately, comfort foods are typically loaded with carbs, sugar, and grains by nature, and when you're trying to eat more healthily, it can be tough to replicate these dishes in a way that fits your lifestyle. With *Keto Comfort Foods*, you'll find classic dishes that don't compromise flavor, texture, or the ability to satisfy. No more sacrificing your favorite meals!

Inside you'll find one hundred keto-friendly comfort foods to satisfy your cravings and remind you of home, all while staying on track. You'll also find a list of low-carb swaps to use as a guide for replacing some of those heavier items.

The key to enjoying comfort foods on the ketogenic diet is to make smart substitutions. You'll soon realize that you don't need traditional breads, noodles, or flours to create those amazing, classic comfort dishes. It can all be done in a way that makes you feel great and even helps you lose weight.

Whether you're looking to stabilize your blood sugar levels or lose body fat, *Keto Comfort Foods* is full of mouthwatering recipes that will allow you to indulge your cravings without losing sight of your keto diet goals.

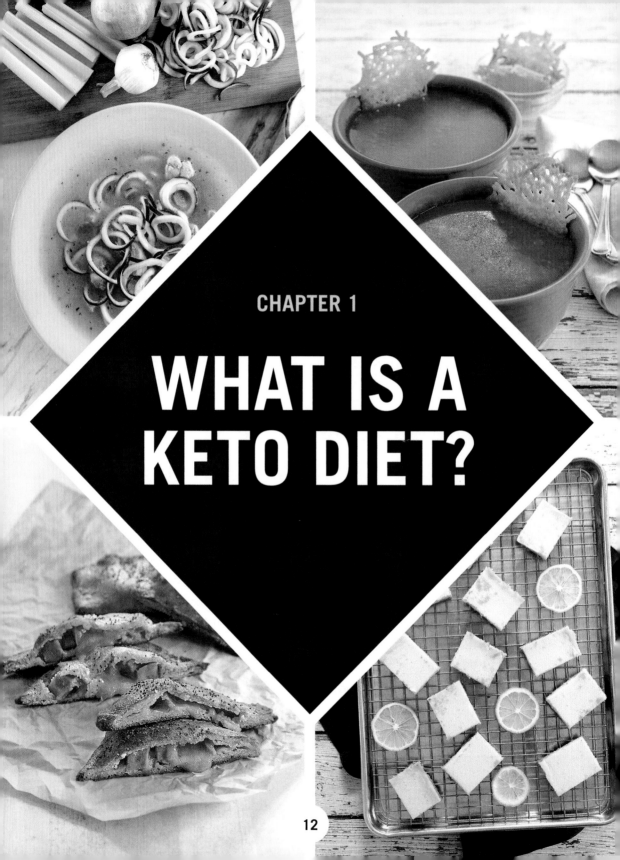

CHAPTER 1

WHAT IS A KETO DIET?

When you eat a very high-carb diet (consuming a lot of pizza, pasta, and bread, for example) your body takes those carbs and turns them into glucose to power itself. Eating more carbs than your body needs, however, can lead to potential health problems, such as weight gain, mood swings, lethargy, and cravings. The keto diet aims to minimize carb consumption.

THE KETO DIET, EXPLAINED

The ketogenic, or keto, diet is a very low-carb, moderate-protein, and high-fat diet that allows the body to fuel itself without the use of glucose or high levels of carbohydrates. When you cut out the carbs, your metabolism burns fat instead.

When the body is in short supply of glucose, ketones are made in the liver from the breakdown of fats through a process called *ketosis*. It's important to note that ketosis differs greatly from ketoacidosis, which is a serious medical condition caused by dangerously high levels of ketones in those with type 1 diabetes.

With careful tracking, creative meals, and self-control, this diet can lead to weight loss, lower blood sugar, regulated insulin levels, and controlled cravings.

WHAT ARE MACROS?

Macronutrients, or macros, are what make up the caloric content of food. All food falls into the categories of carbohydrates, protein, and fat. When you're following a keto lifestyle, it is very important to track how many grams of each macronutrient you consume each day.

- Carbs should provide around 5 percent of your daily calories
- Proteins should provide around 25 percent of your daily calories
- Healthy fats should provide around 70 percent of your daily calories

Calculating how many grams of each macro you want to eat ahead of time will help you plan your meals and snacks in a way that will fill you up and meet your goals.

Carbs

Typically, a ketogenic diet restricts carbs to 0–50 grams per day. Most people following the keto diet opt to track net carbs instead of total carbs. In a pinch, you can use this equation to calculate net carbs:

Total carbs – dietary fiber = net carbs

The net carb totals in this book are calculated using a more precise formula that factors in the effect of certain sugar alcohols. Tracking net carbs is generally the preferred method because of how your body reacts to the fiber and sugar alcohols. On nutrition labels, the grams of dietary fiber and sugar alcohols are already included in the total carb count, but because fiber and (some) sugar alcohols are carbs that your body can't digest, they have no effect on your blood sugar levels and can be subtracted.

Careful planning is key to helping you feel less restricted. For example, you may choose to enjoy a dish that is 10 grams of net carbs. While some may think that is too much for a single meal, it's perfectly fine as long as you keep track of the carbs you're eating for the rest of the day to stay within your goals. You may choose to eat very few carbs throughout the day so you can enjoy a higher-carb snack in the evening, such as mixed berries and a square of low-carb chocolate. Try to look at your day as a whole and decide how you would like to utilize each of your macronutrients.

Protein

Protein is essential for muscle building and muscle retaining. If you're losing weight, a careful check to be sure you're eating enough proteins helps ensure that your body is not also losing muscle. An adequate amount of proteins, usually obtained from sources such as meat, fish, and eggs, helps your body feel fuller and discourages overeating.

Fats

Some of the best-quality fats come from natural sources such as fish, avocados, and nuts. These fats may help reduce your cholesterol, keep your heart strong, and fuel your body throughout the day.

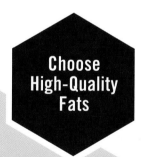

Choose High-Quality Fats

Just because keto is a high-fat diet, it doesn't mean you're free to eat all the fats you want. You should always beware of unhealthy fats, however, that can come from foods like cookies and French fries. Overconsumption of these, especially in conjunction with a high-carb diet, can contribute to heart disease, low energy, and unwanted weight gain. Fat has the highest amount of calories per gram, and you can easily go overboard and gain weight if you're not careful.

It's helpful to think of "high fat" in terms of a percentage of your calories. If carbs represent 5 percent of your calorie consumption and protein is roughly 25 percent, then the remaining 70 percent is fat (these numbers are just examples). That 70 percent can look very different for different people depending on their caloric intake. For some it may be 70 grams of fat, and for others it may be 150 grams. This is why it's helpful to calculate your macros.

Regulating Your Macros

When considering how much of each macro you're eating, think about these tips:

- **Carbs are a limit:** Don't go above your allotted daily net carbs.
- **Protein is a goal:** This is the most important macro to hit. If you're losing weight, you want to make sure you're eating enough protein to keep you from also losing muscle.
- **Fat is a lever:** In this diet, fat is designed to keep you full. If you're hungry, go ahead and eat that healthy fat up to your limit. If you're not hungry, you don't have to hit your fat macros.

With the quick, easy, and hearty recipes in this book, you should never feel deprived on your keto journey just because you're reducing your carb consumption. Just remember, if you slip up, the most important thing is to get back on track as quickly as possible. Allow yourself grace and time, but never give up just because you slipped up.

STAYING IN KETOSIS

Reducing your carb consumption will help you stay in ketosis. Remember, ketosis is a metabolic state, not the food you eat. Because of this, it's generally accepted that there are not "keto foods" and "non-keto foods." That said, some very high-carb foods just will not work with the diet based on your goal amount of carbohydrates. Most people following the keto diet keep their net carbs under 20 grams per day. This loose guide is generally accepted as a safe zone for staying in ketosis, though according to your specific goals and exercise habits, you may be able to go higher or lower.

The Role Fat Plays in Ketosis

A common misconception is that the amount of fat you consume on the keto diet dictates the depth of ketosis you're in. The state of ketosis is achieved by the amount of carbs you restrict rather than the amount of fat you ingest. Think of your fat macro as a filler. You've calculated how much protein your muscles need (using an online calculator) and decided on your amount of carbohydrates, and the final piece of the puzzle is your fat intake.

Testing Your Ketone Levels

If you're tracking your macros in a nutrition app, there's not much need for testing your ketone levels, but it can be a helpful tool for beginners or those who like to experiment with their body's limits. The two main types of testing methods are urine strips and blood ketone meters.

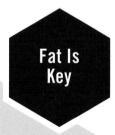

Fat Is Key

If you were to eat only protein and carbs, your calories wouldn't be enough to sustain you, which is why fat is important. It's a less rigid macro than protein because if you're feeling a little less hungry, it's usually okay to not meet your fat grams for the day, as long as you're careful to not severely and con-sistently undereat.

- **Urine strips** are easily attainable and inexpensive. They will give you a good idea of if you're on the right track. The best approach to these strips isn't to worry if you're in the darkest purple area but to simply see if your body is producing excess ketones. The ketone range can vary based on the time of day, your hydration level, and the sensitivity of the test. It may take a few days for your body to begin producing ke-tones, but once it does, you can toss the strips or test intermittently.

- **Blood ketone meters** are generally more expensive, but they are more accurate and report your ketone levels numerically.

If you want to gauge your body's reaction to different sweeteners, products, or carb amounts, these tests can be good tools.

LOW-CARB SWAPS

Smart substitutions are the key to success with a keto lifestyle. Here is a list of the most common high-carb foods you will likely be looking to replace on a ketogenic diet. Their substitutions are much lower in carb counts, but are just as satisfying!

Ingredient	Keto Substitution
All-purpose flour	Almond flour, coconut flour
Rice	Cauliflower rice (Chapter 5)
Potatoes	Cauliflower, jicamas, radishes
Bread crumbs	Crushed pork rinds, crushed cheese crisps
Pasta	Zucchini noodles, spaghetti squash, shredded cabbage, shirataki noodles
Sugar	Erythritol, monk fruit, stevia
Chocolate	Sugar-free chocolate (try Lily's Sweets or ChocZero) (avoid the ingredient maltitol)
Milk	Unsweetened almond milk, unsweetened coconut milk
Ice cream	Mason Jar Vanilla Ice Cream (Chapter 8), Rebel Creamery

HELPFUL TIPS FOR STARTING KETO

As you begin embracing the keto lifestyle, think about these tips to help you start off on the right foot and stay on track, even if you slip up once in a while.

Calculate Your Macros

Everybody does keto a little differently because everyone has different goals and reasons for starting the diet. It's important to use an online calculator to determine your macronutrient goals so you can reach your goals most effectively. Calculating your macros can also help you have a better understanding of the nutritional value of the foods you're eating.

Start Slowly If You Need To

While some might be able to toss the bread and never look back, you might not be ready to completely ditch the carbs. Just as there's no one way to approach the keto diet, there's no one way to start. You could try one of these methods to ease in:

- Experiment to see what one day of keto-friendly eating would look like, followed by one week before fully committing.
- Ditch all *added* sugars.
- Avoid eating bread.

Sometimes when making a big adjustment, a slow transition leads to a more sustainable and long-lasting change, so don't be afraid to take your time.

Learn to Read Nutrition Labels

In order to effectively maintain your keto diet, you'll need to become very familiar with nutrition labels. Make a habit out of checking the labels of everything you pick up at the store. Calories are important to consider, especially if you're doing the keto diet for weight loss. You'll also want to keep a close eye on total carbohydrates, dietary fiber, protein, and fat. These are the essential markers to figuring out if a food item is a good fit for your diet.

Skip Low-Fat Dairy Products

Keep in mind that you should not eat much, if any, low- and reduced-fat dairy products while following the keto diet. They usually contain far more carbs and sugar than the full-fat versions.

Another important tip to remember is that even though some brands may advertise their products as having 0 grams of total carbohydrates per serving, that is often because they are allowed to round that number down to 0. For example, all heavy whipping creams have carbs, typically about 0.4 grams per tablespoon. Most brands you'll pick up in the grocery store will indicate 0 grams per serving, but that number is rounded down. (All dairy has carbs!) Without that knowledge you could easily be taking in way more carbs than you intended. One cup of heavy whipping cream in a recipe will add 6.4 grams of carbs to your dish, a significant difference from the 0 grams that you might have expected. You don't need to worry too much about the exact amounts; just be mindful that rounding often happens in labeling.

Stick to Whole Foods As Much As Possible

With the increased popularity of the keto diet, it's easy to find a lot of premade keto-friendly products in your local grocery store. As you may expect, not all of these products are trustworthy. Some use sweeteners that are low in carbs, but they may cause blood sugar spikes, they may irritate your stomach from low-quality sweeteners or excessive fiber, or they just won't fill you up.

LET'S GET STARTED

Learning to navigate your new way of eating can be exciting. Encourage yourself to try new vegetables, learn to cook new cuts of meat, and experiment with new spices and herbs that elevate the flavor of your dishes.

Now that you have a better understanding of the ketogenic diet, let's get cooking! You'll find plenty of recipes to comfort all ages and suit all tastes. Each recipe includes approximate prep and cook times so you can plan your schedule accordingly. Use these recipes as a guide and always feel free to season intuitively and customize dishes to your liking.

Better Choices Lead to Better Outcomes

It's usually a wise choice to pick whole foods instead of heavily processed foods when possible, especially when you're starting out. A protein bar may be delicious, but a lemon butter chicken thigh with crispy skin has fewer ingredients and can be even more satisfying. Choosing whole foods makes sure you're nourishing your body and helps keep your carb-heavy cravings at bay.

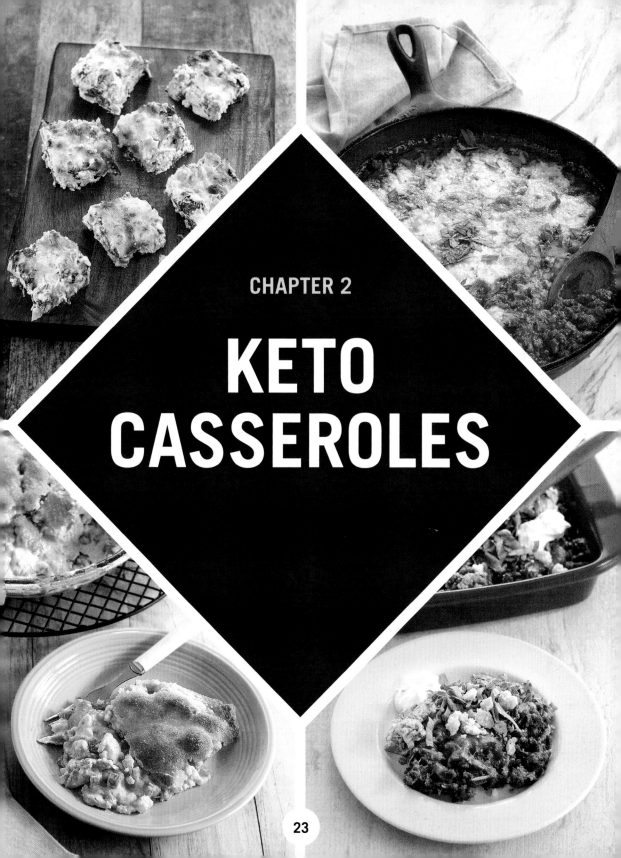

CHAPTER 2

KETO CASSEROLES

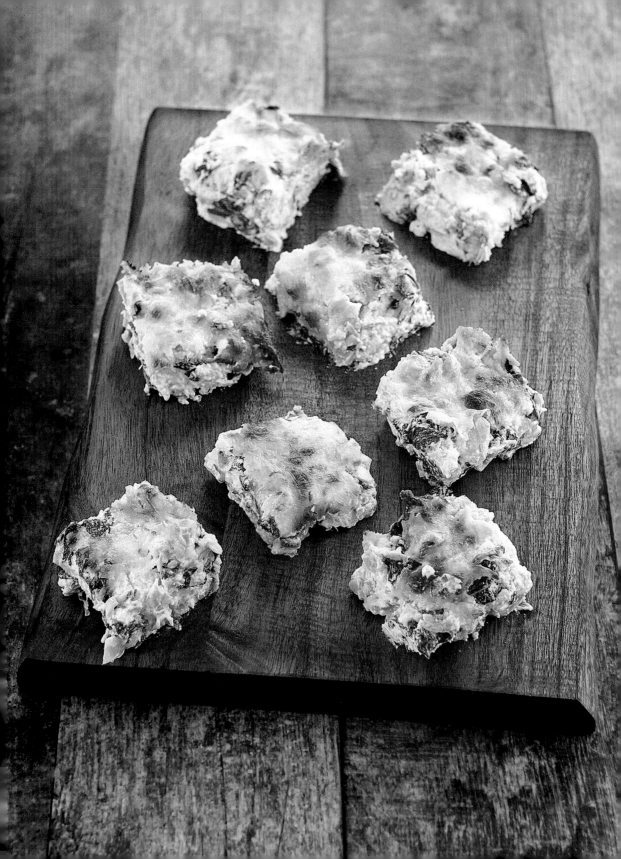

SPINACH ARTICHOKE CHICKEN CASSEROLE

If you're a fan of the dip, you'll love this ultracreamy dish! The rich cheese sauce made without any flour or traditional carb-filled thickeners comes together in just minutes. This recipe calls for chicken that's already cooked, which makes it a great option for using up leftovers. If you don't have leftovers, you can also grab a rotisserie chicken at the grocery store instead.

Prep time 10 minutes | **Cook time** 30 minutes | **Serves 6**

1 tablespoon salted butter

2 tablespoons diced peeled red onion

2 cups fresh spinach

1 (14-ounce) can artichoke hearts, drained and chopped

8 ounces cream cheese, softened

½ cup mayonnaise

⅓ cup sour cream

¼ teaspoon garlic powder

3 cups cubed cooked boneless, skinless chicken breast

1 cup shredded mozzarella, divided

¼ cup shredded Parmesan

Per Serving

Calories: 514 | Fat: 36g | Protein: 32g | Sodium: 630mg | Fiber: 3g | Carbohydrates: 9g | Net Carbohydrates: 6g | Sugar: 2g

1 Preheat the oven to 400°F.

2 In a large skillet over medium heat, melt butter. Add onion to the pan and sauté until it begins to soften, about 2–3 minutes.

3 Add spinach and artichokes. Continue cooking until spinach is wilted, about 4–5 minutes.

4 In a large bowl, mix cream cheese, mayonnaise, sour cream, and garlic powder until smooth. Add this mixture to the pan and stir carefully until all the ingredients are combined, about 30 seconds.

5 Add chicken, ¾ cup mozzarella, and Parmesan to the pan and stir until combined, about 30 seconds.

6 Place the mixture into an 8" × 8" baking dish and top with the remaining mozzarella. Bake for 20 minutes or until the top begins to turn golden brown and bubbles around the edges. Serve warm.

EASY CHICKEN AND RICE CASSEROLE

This dish may sound simple, but building complementary flavors can be one of the hardest things to master when you aren't grabbing premade ingredients. Most casseroles use condensed soups, but those are filled with unsavory ingredients that can knock you out of ketosis. Making your own sauce can be very quick and will get your casserole on the table in just over 30 minutes, so don't be intimidated!

Prep time 10 minutes | **Cook time** 25 minutes | **Serves 6**

1 (12-ounce) steamer bag cauliflower rice

2 tablespoons salted butter, melted

¼ medium yellow onion, peeled and finely chopped

3 cups cubed cooked boneless, skinless chicken breast

2 large egg yolks

¼ cup heavy whipping cream

2 ounces cream cheese, softened

1 cup shredded sharp Cheddar

Per Serving
Calories: 358 | Fat: 21g | Protein: 31g | Sodium: 246mg | Fiber: 1g | Carbohydrates: 4g | Net Carbohydrates: 3g | Sugar: 2g

1 Preheat the oven to 400°F.

2 Steam cauliflower rice according to the instructions on the bag. When finished cooking, open the bag to release the steam and set aside.

3 In a large bowl, add butter, onion, and chicken. In a medium bowl, whisk egg yolks, heavy whipping cream, and cream cheese. Mix in Cheddar, then pour the mixture into the large bowl.

4 Stir the ingredients until all chicken pieces are coated in the liquid mixture. Add cauliflower rice, carefully folding into the mixture until just combined.

5 Transfer the mixture into an 8" × 8" casserole dish. Bake for 20 minutes until center is firm and top is golden. Allow to cool for 10 minutes. Serve warm.

Weeknight Win!

This dish uses shortcuts such as a vegetable steamer bag to save you time. Grab a rotisserie chicken at the store so you're ready to make this comforting and nutritious meal any day of the week. If you love meal prepping, feel free to use fresh cauliflower rice and chicken if you prefer.

CHICKEN PARMESAN CASSEROLE

Traditionally, this dish can take a while to make, but this easy low-carb version is ready much faster and has far fewer carbs. The chicken isn't breaded, but it has a crunchy topping made of cheese that will have you wondering how you ever went without it. The zucchini adds a noodle feel, like a pasta dish you might order in a restaurant, but feel free to leave it out.

Prep time 10 minutes | **Cook time** 35 minutes | **Serves 4**

2 tablespoons salted butter
1 tablespoon olive oil
½ teaspoon dried basil
¼ teaspoon dried oregano
⅛ teaspoon garlic powder
1½ pounds boneless, skinless chicken thigh
1½ cups low-carb marinara sauce
1 medium zucchini, grated
2 ounces fresh mini mozzarella balls
½ cup shredded mozzarella
½ cup grated Parmesan
2 ounces 100% Parmesan cheese crisps, crushed

Per Serving
Calories: 537 | Fat: 33g | Protein: 43g | Sodium: 1,023mg | Fiber: 1g | Carbohydrates: 9g | Net Carbohydrates: 8g | Sugar: 5g

1 Preheat the oven to 400°F.

2 In a medium skillet over medium heat, warm butter and olive oil. Sprinkle basil, oregano, and garlic powder evenly on both sides of chicken.

3 Place chicken into the skillet and let cook for about 7 minutes on each side until no pink remains and the internal temperature is at least 165°F. Let cool for 3 minutes, then chop into bite-sized pieces.

4 Place chicken in the bottom of an 8" × 8" baking dish. Pour marinara sauce over chicken and toss to coat.

5 Place zucchini shreds into a kitchen towel or cheese-cloth to remove the excess moisture, then sprinkle the zucchini on top of the sauce. Scatter mozzarella balls on top and toss to coat everything. Sprinkle the top with shredded mozzarella, Parmesan, and cheese crisps.

6 Bake for 20 minutes or until cheese is melted and golden. Let cool for 10 minutes. Serve warm.

Low-Carb Marinara Sauce

There is a growing number of great options for low-sugar sauces that you can choose from if you prefer not to make your own. Tomatoes do have natural sugar, so don't expect to see any labels with 0 grams of sugar, but try to keep it under 5 grams of carbs per serving and avoid added sugars. Rao's brand is a great low-carb option and can likely be found next to the regular sauces at your local grocery store.

CHEESY BROCCOLI AND CAULIFLOWER CASSEROLE

Eating your vegetables couldn't be tastier than it is with this delicious casserole! If you struggle to feed picky eaters, adding a creamy cheese sauce can make vegetables a lot more enjoyable. Vegetables are an important part of any diet because they provide essential vitamins and minerals. Feel free to add your favorite protein to this dish to make it even heartier.

Prep time 10 minutes | **Cook time** 35 minutes | **Serves 4**

2 medium broccoli crowns, stems removed and cut into small florets

1 medium head cauliflower, leaves removed, cored, and cut into small florets

4 tablespoons salted butter

¼ medium yellow onion, peeled and chopped

1 clove garlic, peeled and finely minced

2 ounces cream cheese, softened

½ cup heavy whipping cream

1½ cups shredded sharp Cheddar

⅛ teaspoon ground black pepper

Per Serving
Calories: 568 | Fat: 38g | Protein: 23g | Sodium: 571mg | Fiber: 11g | Carbohydrates: 30g | Net Carbohydrates: 19g | Sugar: 10g

1 Preheat the oven to 350°F.

2 In a large pot over medium heat, bring 2 cups water to a boil. Put broccoli and cauliflower into a steamer basket and carefully lower it into the water. Cover pot and allow vegetables to steam for 7 minutes.

3 In a medium skillet over medium heat, melt butter. Add onion and sauté until it begins to soften, about 3 minutes. Add garlic, cream cheese, and heavy whipping cream, whisking until smooth, about 2 minutes.

4 Turn off the heat and add Cheddar, whisking until smooth, about 2 minutes. Sprinkle with pepper.

5 Place steamed vegetables in a 9" × 9" baking dish and pour the cheese sauce over them. Use a spoon to gently coat the vegetables with cheese and press into a flat layer.

6 Bake for 20 minutes or until the top and edges begin to brown, and the mixture is bubbling. Let cool for 5 minutes. Serve warm.

CHICKEN CORDON BLEU CASSEROLE

This dish remakes the breaded carb-filled version with keto-friendly ingredients, and it still has that crunch you enjoy! The creamy sauce has a little tang, which adds another dimension to the flavors. The cheese sauce takes just a couple minutes to make but is guaranteed to be your family's favorite part!

Prep time 15 minutes | **Cook time** 35 minutes | **Serves 6**

2 tablespoons coconut oil

1 pound boneless, skinless chicken thigh

⅛ teaspoon finely ground sea salt

¼ teaspoon ground black pepper

2 cups diced cooked ham

2 tablespoons Dijon mustard

4 tablespoons salted butter

4 tablespoons cream cheese, softened

¾ cup heavy whipping cream

¼ cup chicken broth

1 cup shredded Swiss cheese

1 cup shredded Monterey jack, divided

2 ounces plain pork rinds, crushed

Per Serving
Calories: 615 | Fat: 46g | Protein: 40g | Sodium: 1,285mg | Fiber: 0g | Carbohydrates: 3g | Net Carbohydrates: 3g | Sugar: 2g

1 Preheat the oven to 400°F.

2 In a medium skillet over medium heat, melt coconut oil. Place chicken into the skillet and sprinkle both sides with salt and pepper. Cook for 7 minutes per side or until no pink remains and the internal temperature is at least 165°F.

3 Chop chicken into bite-sized pieces and place in an 8" × 8" baking dish. Add ham and mustard and toss.

4 In a medium saucepan over medium heat, melt butter. Whisk in cream cheese, heavy whipping cream, and broth. Sprinkle in Swiss cheese and whisk until smooth. Add ½ cup Monterey jack, whisking until smooth, about 1 minute.

5 Pour the cheese sauce into the baking dish and toss with meat until fully coated. Sprinkle the top with the remaining Monterey jack and pork rinds.

6 Bake for 20 minutes or until bubbling and the top is golden brown. Let cool for 10 minutes before serving.

Don't Like Pork Rinds?

Pork rinds are used as a dipper, casserole topping, and even breading in many keto recipes. They're high fat and get crispy so they're a perfect substitution for flour. If you don't like them, just leave them out or swap in crushed 100 percent cheese crisps instead.

SKILLET LASAGNA

This baked lasagna ditches the noodles to bring the savory Italian flavors of the dish to the forefront. The two types of meat add bulk to the meal, so it's just as filling as its "carby" counterpart. The cheese mixture adds that classic lasagna taste to this dish, but if you don't like ricotta, simply swap it out with full-fat cottage cheese to keep that creamy taste. To add a big crunch, feel free to top with crushed cheese crisps or crushed pork rinds!

Prep time 20 minutes | **Cook time** 45 minutes | **Serves 6**

1 pound 80/20 ground beef

½ pound Italian ground sausage

¼ cup chopped peeled white onion

1½ cups low-carb marinara sauce

1 teaspoon dried oregano, divided

¾ teaspoon garlic powder, divided

½ cup ricotta

1 cup shredded mozzarella, divided

⅔ cup Parmesan, divided

2 tablespoons chopped fresh parsley

Per Serving

Calories: 374 | Fat: 23g | Protein: 28g | Sodium: 540mg | Fiber: 1g | Carbohydrates: 9g | Net Carbohydrates: 8g | Sugar: 3g

1 Preheat the oven to 400°F.

2 In a 12" cast-iron skillet (or other oven-safe equivalent) over medium heat, brown ground beef and sausage over medium heat until no pink remains, about 15 minutes. Drain the excess fat and return to heat.

3 Add onion to the pan and sauté with meat until onion begins to soften, about 3 minutes. Add marinara sauce, ½ teaspoon oregano, and ½ teaspoon garlic powder and allow to simmer for 5 minutes.

4 In a medium bowl, mix ricotta, ½ cup mozzarella, ⅓ cup Parmesan, and the remaining oregano and garlic powder until combined.

5 Turn off the heat and spread the meat around the pan to form an even layer. Place spoonfuls of the cheese mixture on top of the meat mixture, pushing them down with the spoon to the bottom of the pan.

6 Sprinkle the top with the remaining mozzarella and Parmesan. Bake for 20 minutes until bubbling and the top begins to turn golden. Garnish with parsley. Serve warm.

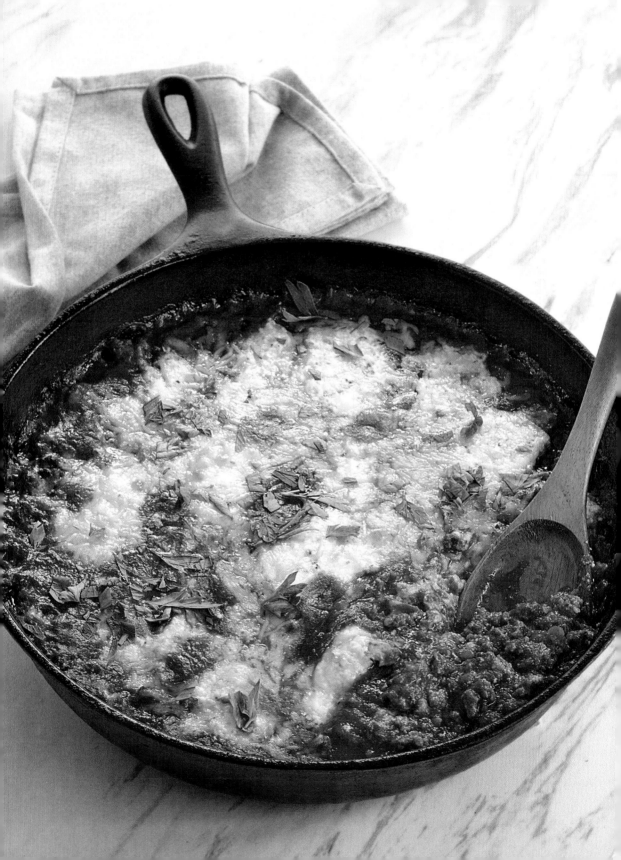

PHILLY CHEESESTEAK CASSEROLE

If you loved these sandwiches in your carb-eating days, you'll be glad to learn you can still enjoy all their flavors in keto form! Not only is this dish easy to prepare, but it's also a warm comfort food at its finest. It's filled with flavorful meat, a rich cheese sauce, and even some vegetables for extra nutrients. When your plate is piled high with a delicious scoop, you'll wonder why you ever let bread get in the way of the real flavors!

Prep time 10 minutes | **Cook time** 30 minutes | **Serves 6**

2 tablespoons coconut oil

1½ pounds thinly sliced rib eye

⅛ teaspoon finely ground pink Himalayan salt

¼ teaspoon ground black pepper

1 medium green bell pepper, seeded and thinly sliced

¼ medium white onion, peeled and thinly sliced

4 tablespoons salted butter

4 ounces cream cheese, softened

¾ cup heavy whipping cream

5 (⅔-ounce, medium-thick) slices provolone, chopped

1 cup shredded Monterey jack, divided

1 Preheat the oven to 400°F.

2 In a large skillet over medium heat, melt coconut oil. Sear rib eye and sprinkle with salt and black pepper. When no pink remains in rib eye, about 7 minutes, remove meat and place into a 9" × 9" baking dish. Add bell pepper and onion and toss.

3 In the same large skillet over medium heat, melt butter. Whisk in cream cheese and heavy whipping cream until smooth, about 30 seconds.

4 Whisk in provolone and ½ cup Monterey jack until smooth, about 1 minute. Pour the mixture over the meat and vegetables and gently toss until completely covered. Sprinkle the remaining Monterey jack on top and bake for 20 minutes until bubbling and golden brown on top. Cool for 10 minutes, then serve warm.

Per Serving

Calories: 721 | Fat: 60g | Protein: 35g | Sodium: 545mg | Fiber: 0g | Carbohydrates: 4g | Net Carbohydrates: 4g | Sugar: 2g

CAULI-TOT CASSEROLE

Tater Tot Casserole is a midwestern classic that warms many bellies on cold nights. The dish typically uses cream of mushroom soup, which is loaded with carbs. To make a thickener in a keto-friendly way, just grab a few ingredients and make it yourself. You'll replace traditional Tater Tots with a lower-carb version made from cauliflower. This dish does take a little longer to prepare than some others, but the end result is so delicious that it's worth it.

Prep time 20 minutes | **Cook time** 50 minutes | **Serves 6**

2 (12-ounce) steamer bags cauliflower florets

½ cup shredded mozzarella

2 ounces plain pork rinds, finely ground

1 large egg

1 pound 80/20 ground beef

4 tablespoons salted butter

½ cup chopped cremini mushrooms

¼ medium yellow onion, peeled and chopped

1 clove garlic, peeled and finely minced

½ cup vegetable broth

½ cup heavy whipping cream

⅛ teaspoon ground black pepper

¼ teaspoon finely ground pink Himalayan salt

¼ teaspoon xanthan gum

¾ cup shredded mild Cheddar

Per Serving

Calories: 460 | Fat: 32g | Protein: 29g | Sodium: 562mg | Fiber: 3g | Carbohydrates: 8g | Net Carbohydrates: 5g | Sugar: 4g

1 Preheat the oven to 400°F. Line a large baking sheet with parchment paper.

2 Place the cauliflower bags into the microwave and cook according to the package directions. Remove and place into a food processor.

3 Add mozzarella, pork rinds, and egg to the food processor. Pulse for 30–45 seconds until the mixture is smooth.

4 Use a tablespoon to scoop out a round of dough and form into about twenty Tater Tot shapes. Place onto the prepared baking sheet. Bake for 15 minutes, flipping halfway through, until golden brown.

5 In a medium skillet over medium heat, brown ground beef until no pink remains, about 10 minutes. Drain the excess grease and return the skillet to the stovetop. Add butter and let melt, then add mushrooms and onion. Sauté for 3 minutes or until vegetables begin to soften.

6 Add garlic to the pan and sauté for 30 seconds, then pour in broth. Bring the mixture to a boil, then reduce the heat to a simmer for 10 minutes.

7 Pour in heavy whipping cream and sprinkle with pepper, salt, and xanthan gum. Allow about 2 minutes to thicken, then remove from heat and pour into a 9" × 9" baking dish.

8 Place the prepared cauliflower around the top, then sprinkle with Cheddar. Bake for 15 minutes or until cheese is melted and the mixture is bubbling. Allow 10 minutes to cool before serving.

BREAKFAST CASSEROLE

This casserole has two kinds of meat and fluffy eggs, so you will satisfy not only your eyes but also your taste buds. The jicama adds a texture similar to hash browns. This is a great dish to make for family get-togethers to show off how delicious following a low-carb lifestyle can truly be!

Prep time 15 minutes | **Cook time** 35 minutes | **Serves 6**

1 pound ground pork breakfast sausage
4 tablespoons salted butter
6 large eggs
¼ cup heavy whipping cream
½ cup shredded Monterey jack
2 cups diced cooked ham
1 cup peeled and grated jicama
½ cup shredded mild Cheddar

Per Serving
Calories: 527 | Fat: 39g | Protein: 33g | Sodium: 946mg | Fiber: 1g | Carbohydrates: 4g | Net Carbohydrates: 3g | Sugar: 1g

1 Preheat the oven to 350°F.

2 In a medium skillet over medium heat, cook sausage until no pink remains, about 12 minutes. Drain the excess grease and set meat aside.

3 In a clean medium skillet over medium heat, melt butter. Crack eggs open into the pan and whisk together with heavy whipping cream.

4 Cook the egg mixture for 4–6 minutes, stirring occasionally until eggs are soft and scrambled but still a little runny. They will finish cooking in the oven.

5 Stir in Monterey jack, ham, jicama, and cooked sausage until combined. Pour the mixture into an 8" × 8" baking dish. Top with Cheddar and bake for 17 minutes or until cheese is melted and golden brown. Serve warm.

What Is Jicama?

Jicama is a starchy, sweet, potato-like vegetable. When cooked, it has the texture of a potato, which makes it a great addition to this dish. It has more carbs than cauliflower has, for example, but it can be a nice alternative to potatoes in small amounts.

SLOPPY JOE CASSEROLE

This recipe might remind you of an open-faced sandwich, except the bread is on the top. The bottom part of this casserole tastes like the traditional dish, but it is made with tomato paste instead of tomato purée because it has fewer carbs. The biscuits on top are golden and crispy—the perfect complement to this tangy beef dish!

Prep time 10 minutes | **Cook time** 45 minutes | **Serves 4**

1 pound 80/20 ground beef

2 tablespoons salted butter

½ medium yellow onion, peeled and diced

1 medium green bell pepper, seeded and chopped

1 tablespoon tomato paste

2 teaspoons granular erythritol

½ cup chicken broth

¼ cup low-carb ketchup

½ teaspoon chili powder

1 teaspoon yellow mustard

1 teaspoon Worcestershire sauce

1¼ cups finely ground blanched almond flour

1½ cups shredded mozzarella

4 tablespoons salted butter, cubed

1 teaspoon baking powder

½ teaspoon apple cider vinegar

Per Serving

Calories: 472 | Fat: 35g | Protein: 25g | Sodium: 590mg | Fiber: 3g | Carbohydrates: 11g | Sugar Alcohol: 1g | Net Carbohydrates: 8g | Sugar: 4g

1 Preheat the oven to 400°F.

2 In a large skillet over medium heat, brown the ground beef until no pink remains, about 10 minutes. Drain the excess grease from the pan, then return the pan to medium heat.

3 Add 2 tablespoons butter, onion, and bell pepper to the pan. Cook for 3 minutes or until vegetables begin to soften.

4 Whisk in tomato paste, erythritol, broth, and ketchup until combined, about 30 seconds.

5 Sprinkle in chili powder, then whisk in mustard and Worcestershire sauce. Cook for 10 minutes, stirring occasionally, then pour into an 8" × 8" casserole dish.

6 In a large microwave-safe bowl, mix almond flour, mozzarella, and cubed butter. Microwave for 45 seconds, then stir. Microwave for an additional 15 seconds, then add baking powder and vinegar and stir until a soft ball forms. Cut the dough into six pieces and form into disc shapes. Place them on top of the casserole, then bake for 20 minutes or until golden brown. Let cool for 10 minutes. Serve warm.

Make It More Filling

To make this dish even more filling, add extra meat or vegetables. Cauliflower offers an excellent potato-like texture, plus added nutrients. Or, you could add an extra ½ pound of meat to fill out the dish.

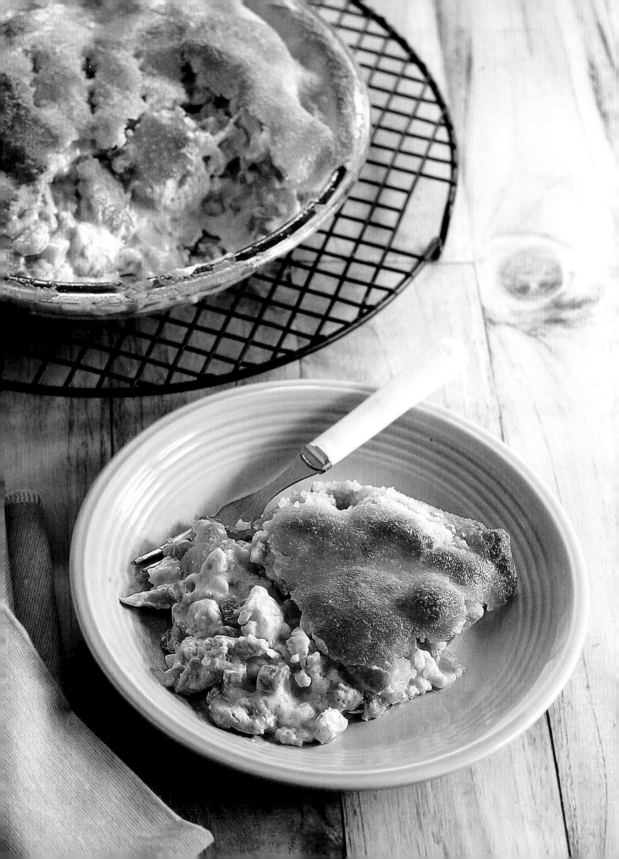

CHICKEN POTPIE CASSEROLE

This recipe is the epitome of comfort food! Though some would consider carrots taboo on a keto diet, feel free to eat them if they can fit into your daily macros. You can leave out carrots to lower the carbs of this dish to better fit your personal needs.

Prep time 10 minutes | **Cook time** 60 minutes | **Serves 6**

2 tablespoons coconut oil

1 pound boneless, skinless chicken thigh

8 tablespoons salted butter, divided

¼ medium yellow onion, peeled and diced

¾ cup chicken broth

½ large carrot, peeled and chopped

1 medium stalk celery, chopped

2 cups chopped cauliflower florets

⅛ teaspoon dried thyme

⅛ teaspoon finely ground pink Himalayan salt

⅛ teaspoon ground black pepper

¼ teaspoon xanthan gum

½ cup heavy whipping cream

2 ounces cream cheese, softened

1½ cups shredded mozzarella

1½ cups finely ground blanched almond flour

1 large egg yolk, whisked for egg wash

Per Serving

Calories: 648 | Fat: 53g | Protein: 28g | Sodium: 479mg | Fiber: 4g | Carbohydrates: 11g | Net Carbohydrates: 7g | Sugar: 4g

1 Preheat the oven to 400°F.

2 In a medium skillet over medium heat, melt coconut oil. Cook chicken until no pink remains and internal temperature is at least 165°F, about 7 minutes per side. Place on a cutting board to cool for about 5 minutes, then cut into bite-sized pieces.

3 In a medium pot over medium heat, melt 4 tablespoons butter. Add onion and sauté 3 minutes or until soft and fragrant. Pour in chicken broth and add carrot, celery, cauliflower, thyme, salt, and pepper.

4 Bring the pot to a boil over high heat for 1 minute, then reduce to a simmer, uncovered, for 15 minutes until vegetables soften. Sprinkle xanthan gum in the pot, whisking quickly, then pour in heavy cream. Whisk in cream cheese. Add in the cooked chicken.

5 Turn the heat to low and let the mixture thicken for 10 minutes until thick and creamy.

6 In a large microwave-safe bowl, add mozzarella, remaining butter, and almond flour. Microwave for 45 seconds, then stir. Microwave for an additional 10 seconds, then stir until a soft ball forms.

7 Place the dough between two pieces of parchment paper on a flat surface and roll into a 9" round.

8 Pour the chicken mixture into a round 9" pie dish. Place the dough on top of the dish, pressing the edges into the pie dish. Cut four slits into the dough and brush entire crust with egg yolk.

9 Bake for 15 minutes or until dough is browned. Let cool for 10 minutes. Spoon into bowls and serve warm.

CRUSTLESS QUICHE LORRAINE

This breakfast casserole is so full of savory flavor that you won't even miss the usual crust. The eggs are fluffier and creamier than you would expect with a frittata. With only a few simple ingredients, this filling dish is the perfect meal to prep the night before and pop in the oven when you get up in the morning.

Prep time 15 minutes | **Cook time** 40 minutes | **Serves 6**

2 tablespoons salted butter
½ medium yellow onion, peeled and diced
1 clove garlic, peeled and finely minced
8 slices bacon
6 large eggs
¾ cup heavy whipping cream
½ cup shredded Swiss cheese
½ cup shredded Monterey jack

Per Serving
Calories: 353 | Fat: 29g |
Protein: 17g | Sodium: 403mg |
Fiber: 0g | Carbohydrates: 3g | Net
Carbohydrates: 3g | Sugar: 2g

1 Preheat the oven to 375°F.

2 In a medium skillet over medium heat, melt butter, then add onion and sauté until it begins to caramelize and become fragrant, about 5 minutes. Add garlic and sauté for 30 seconds. Transfer onion and garlic to a large mixing bowl.

3 Replace the pan over the heat and add bacon. Fry until crispy, about 10–12 minutes. Place bacon on paper towels to absorb the excess grease.

4 Crack open eggs into the bowl with the onion and garlic, then pour in heavy whipping cream. Whisk together until fully combined.

5 Crumble bacon into the bowl, then add the cheeses and mix. Pour the mixture into a round 9" pie dish or similarly sized pan. Bake for 20 minutes. When done, the egg mixture should be set but not overly firm. Let cool for 15 minutes before slicing and serving.

Quiche Options

This is a great meal to customize. Adding chopped ham or mushrooms or other vegetables will make this dish a hit at any brunch. In addition, feel free to switch up the cheese with your favorites!

QUICK JALAPEÑO POPPER CASSEROLE

This is a semi-homemade meal, meaning you can pick up a rotisserie chicken and steamer vegetables at the store, then have the whole thing on the table in less than 30 minutes! Try it on a busy weeknight.

Prep time 10 minutes | **Cook time** 25 minutes | **Serves 4**

1 (12-ounce) steamer bag cauliflower florets

4 ounces cream cheese, softened

3 tablespoons sour cream

½ cup sliced pickled jalapeños

1½ cups shredded sharp Cheddar, divided

½ cup chicken broth

6 slices cooked bacon, crumbled

3 cups diced cooked chicken thigh

1 medium stalk green onion, sliced

Per Serving
Calories: 594 | Fat: 37g | Protein: 46g | Sodium: 1,060mg | Fiber: 2g | Carbohydrates: 7g | Net Carbohydrates: 5g | Sugar: 3g

1 Preheat the oven to 400°F.

2 Steam the cauliflower according to package instructions, about 5 minutes. Let cool for 2 minutes then chop into bite-sized pieces.

3 In a large bowl, mix cream cheese, sour cream, jalapeños, 1 cup Cheddar, broth, and bacon.

4 Fold in chicken and cauliflower. Transfer the mixture into a 9" × 9" baking dish. Sprinkle with the remaining Cheddar. Bake for 20 minutes.

5 Garnish with green onion and let cool for 10 minutes. Serve warm.

LAYERED TACO CASSEROLE

This dish is the perfect midweek meal. It's simple and easy to prepare ahead, plus it's full of your burrito-inspired flavors. The best part of this dish is that you can top it any keto way you want. Try creamy avocado or spicy salsa, or feel free to get creative and add your favorites!

Prep time 10 minutes | **Cook time** 40 minutes | **Serves 4**

1 pound 80/20 ground beef

¼ cup water

2 teaspoons chili powder

2 teaspoons ground cumin

¼ teaspoon garlic powder

¼ teaspoon onion powder

⅛ teaspoon dried oregano

⅛ teaspoon ground black pepper

⅛ teaspoon finely ground sea salt

1 (12-ounce) bag cauliflower rice

½ cup salsa

1 cup shredded mild Cheddar

1 cup shredded romaine lettuce

¼ cup mashed avocado

½ cup sour cream

2 ounces Cheddar cheese crisps, crushed

Per Serving
Calories: 530 | Fat: 34g | Protein: 36g | Sodium: 774mg | Fiber: 5g | Carbohydrates: 11g | Net Carbohydrates: 6g | Sugar: 5g

1 Preheat the oven to 400°F.

2 In a large skillet over medium heat, brown ground beef until no pink remains, about 10 minutes. Drain the excess grease and return the pan to medium heat.

3 Add water, chili powder, cumin, garlic powder, onion powder, oregano, pepper, and salt to the pan. Stir until combined, about 1 minute.

4 Add cauliflower rice and reduce the heat to low and simmer for 5 minutes, stirring occasionally, until water is mostly evaporated.

5 Transfer the mixture to an 8" × 8" baking dish.

6 Place spoonfuls of salsa over the beef mixture, then sprinkle with Cheddar. Bake for 20 minutes.

7 Let cool for 15 minutes, then sprinkle lettuce over top. Place spoonfuls of avocado and sour cream around the dish, then top with cheese crisps. Serve warm.

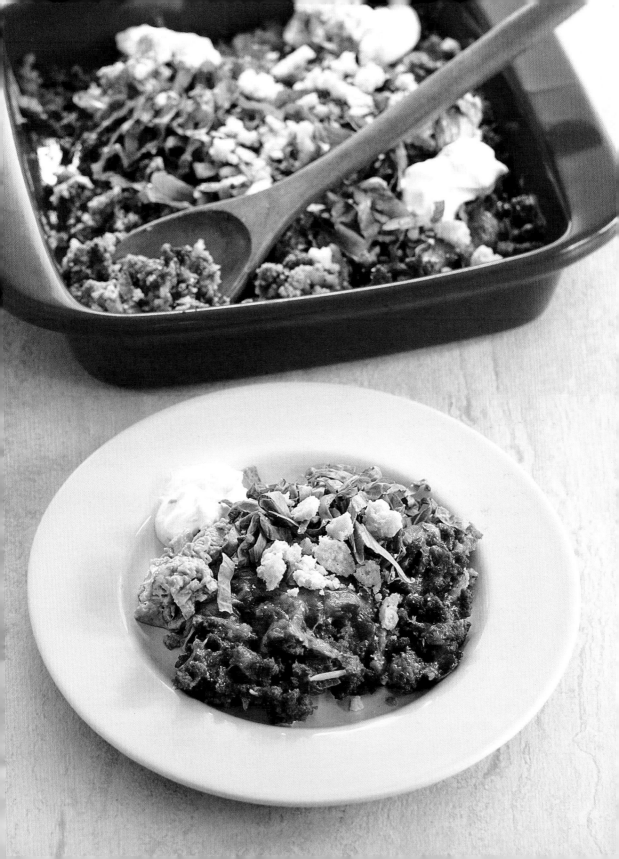

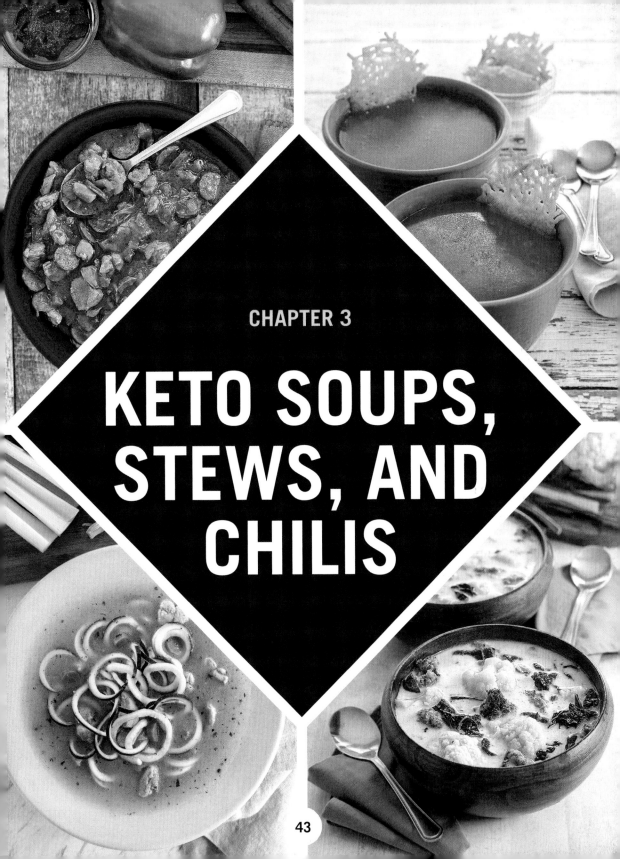

CHAPTER 3

KETO SOUPS, STEWS, AND CHILIS

CINCINNATI-STYLE CHILI

Cincinnati-Style Chili is marked by two unique ingredients: chocolate and noodles. This recipe uses squash for noodles and adds a fresh take on the classic recipe. You can also top it with chopped onion and shredded Cheddar cheese just like the classic dish!

Prep time 10 minutes | **Cook time** 70 minutes | **Serves 6**

2 pounds 80/20 ground beef

2 tablespoons salted butter

½ medium white onion, peeled and chopped

1 (14.5-ounce) can diced tomatoes, drained

4 cups beef broth

¼ cup tomato paste

1 tablespoon hot sauce

½ ounce unsweetened Baker's brand chocolate

½ teaspoon cinnamon

3 tablespoons chili powder

2 teaspoons paprika

1 teaspoon garlic powder

4 medium zucchini, spiralized

Per Serving

Calories: 415 | Fat: 22g | Protein: 34g | Sodium: 1,024mg | Fiber: 5g | Carbohydrates: 14g | Net Carbohydrates: 9g | Sugar: 7g

1 In a large pot over medium heat, brown ground beef until no pink remains, about 10 minutes. Drain the excess grease from the pot and return the pot to medium heat. Add butter, onion, and tomatoes, stirring for 3 minutes until onion becomes fragrant.

2 Pour in broth, then add tomato paste, hot sauce, and chocolate. Stir until tomato paste and chocolate are well incorporated, about 2 minutes, then sprinkle in cinnamon, chili powder, paprika, and garlic powder.

3 Increase the heat to high to allow the chili to come to a boil for 5 minutes. Then cover and reduce the heat to low to simmer for an additional 20 minutes. Uncover and allow to cook down for 30 minutes until thick.

4 Serve over spiralized zucchini.

THREE-MEAT CHILI

Nothing says comfort like a hot bowl of chili during sweater weather. This chunky and flavorful dish will have you forgetting all about those extra carbs from the beans used in traditional recipes. The extra meat makes up for the bulk and will keep you full for hours. Double this batch and freeze the leftovers!

Prep time 15 minutes | **Cook time** 70 minutes | **Serves 6**

1 pound ground sirloin

½ pound ground pork sausage

6 slices bacon, chopped

¼ medium yellow onion, peeled and diced

1 medium green bell pepper, seeded and diced

2 tablespoons tomato paste

1 (14-ounce) can diced tomatoes, drained

2 tablespoons chili powder

1 teaspoon garlic powder

½ teaspoon finely ground pink Himalayan salt

½ teaspoon ground black pepper

5 cups beef broth

1 cup shredded sharp Cheddar

¼ cup sour cream

1 medium stalk green onion

Per Serving
Calories: 373 | Fat: 21g | Protein: 32g | Sodium: 1,443mg | Fiber: 3g | Carbohydrates: 9g | Net Carbohydrates: 6g | Sugar: 4g

1 In a large pot over medium-high heat, brown sirloin, sausage, and bacon until no pink remains, about 12–15 minutes. Drain the excess grease and return the pot to the stove.

2 Add onion, bell pepper, and tomato paste. Stir until combined and let cook for 5 minutes.

3 Pour in tomatoes and sprinkle in chili powder, garlic powder, salt, and black pepper. Pour in broth and cover for 20 minutes to simmer. Remove the lid and stir, then leave uncovered for the remaining 30 minutes to simmer over low heat, stirring occasionally. The liquid will reduce, leaving a thick, chunky chili.

4 Spoon into bowls and top with Cheddar, sour cream, and green onion.

Make It in a Slow Cooker

This recipe makes a great slow-cooker meal! First, cook the meat in a skillet on the stovetop, about 12–15 minutes. Drain the fat and transfer to the slow cooker. Then add the remaining ingredients, except the Cheddar, sour cream, and green onion. Cook on low for 6 hours and leave uncovered for the last hour to thicken.

SPICY WHITE CHICKEN CHILI

This dish is both creamy and spicy—the best of both worlds! In just about an hour you can have a hearty and flavorful meal on the table. You can easily double this comforting meal; freeze it or offer it at a potluck event. For an extra crunch, try topping it with 100 percent cheese crisps, such as ParmCrisps or Whisps.

Prep time 15 minutes | **Cook time** 50 minutes | **Serves 4**

2 tablespoons coconut oil

1 pound boneless, skinless chicken thigh, cubed

¼ medium white onion, peeled and diced

¼ cup seeded and chopped green chilies

1 medium green bell pepper, seeded and chopped

¼ cup pickled jalapeños

4 cups chicken broth

4 ounces cream cheese

¾ cup heavy whipping cream

1 cup shredded Monterey jack

4 tablespoons sour cream

2 tablespoons chopped fresh cilantro

1 In a large pot over medium heat, melt coconut oil. Brown chicken until no pink remains and it reaches an internal temperature of at least 165°F, about 7 minutes per side.

2 Add onion, chilies, bell pepper, and jalapeños to the pan. Cook for 4 minutes until onion and pepper become fragrant, then pour in broth. Let simmer uncovered for 20 minutes.

3 In a small bowl, whisk cream cheese and heavy whipping cream. Whisk the mixture into the pot, then continue cooking for 10 minutes.

4 To serve, top each bowl with ¼ cup cheese, 1 tablespoon sour cream, and 1½ teaspoons cilantro.

Per Serving
Calories: 604 | Fat: 46g | Protein: 31g | Sodium: 1,390mg | Fiber: 1g | Carbohydrates: 7g | Net Carbohydrates: 6g | Sugar: 5g

Not a Fan of Spicy?

If you're not into spicy food, you can still enjoy this dish. Simply swap out the pickled jalapeños for a milder version. Most jars will state whether they are hot or mild. Or you can swap out the pickled jalapeños for serranos.

LOADED "FAUXTATO" SOUP

Cauliflower continues to be the ultimate potato replacement in this hearty and delicious soup. You may appreciate cauliflower's low carb count in comparison to potatoes, but you'll be happy to learn other reasons that it's a better-for-you option: Not only is cauliflower high in fiber; it's also packed with vitamin C! The benefits of this guilt-free vegetable are practically endless!

Prep time 10 minutes | **Cook time** 30 minutes | **Serves 4**

2 tablespoons salted butter

¼ medium white onion, peeled and chopped

1 clove garlic, peeled and finely minced

4 ounces cream cheese, softened

2 (12-ounce) bags frozen cauliflower

5 cups chicken broth

½ cup heavy whipping cream

1 cup shredded sharp Cheddar

4 slices cooked bacon, crumbled

4 tablespoons sour cream

2 medium stalks green onion, sliced

Per Serving

Calories: 500 | Fat: 39g | Protein: 18g | Sodium: 714mg | Fiber: 4g | Carbohydrates: 14g | Net Carbohydrates: 10g | Sugar: 8g

1 In a large pot over medium heat, melt butter. Sauté onion until it begins to soften, about 3 minutes. Then add garlic and sauté for 30 seconds.

2 Add cream cheese and cauliflower to the pot, then pour in chicken broth. Slightly increase the heat to medium-high and bring the soup to a boil. Let boil for 5 minutes, then reduce the heat to low and allow the soup to simmer for 20 minutes or until the cauliflower is tender.

3 Carefully pour the soup into a blender and purée. Pour the soup back into the pot and stir in heavy whipping cream.

4 Top with Cheddar, bacon, sour cream, and green onions. Serve warm.

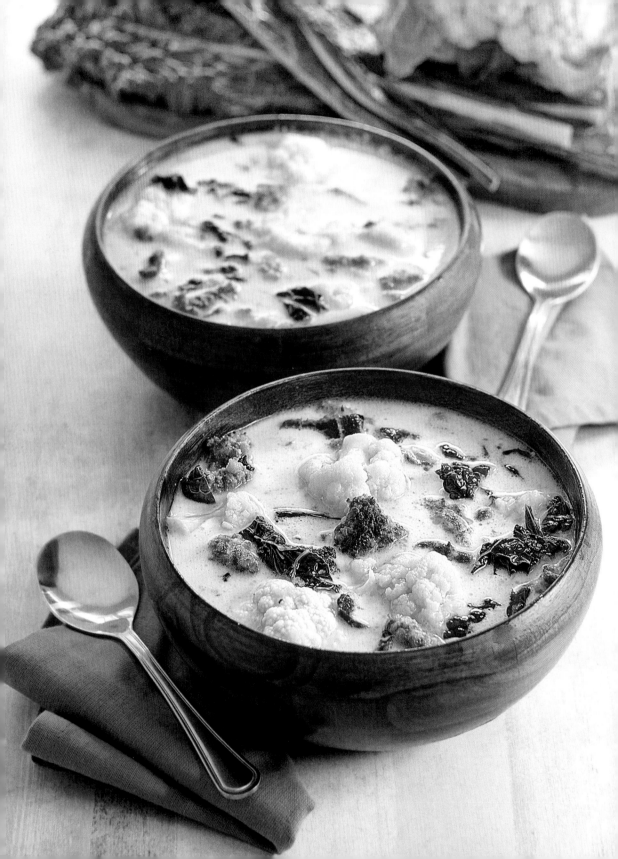

CREAMY TUSCAN SOUP

This rich and creamy soup brings warmth and coziness to any day of the year. You might be surprised that so many soups that seem to be keto-friendly actually use flour as a thickener. For this soup and many others, cream cheese is a great thickener and alternative to using xanthan gum. A low-carb spin on the Italian classic, it's filled with flavorful meats and nutritious vegetables.

Prep time 10 minutes | **Cook time** 60 minutes | **Serves 4**

1 pound ground Italian sausage

4 slices bacon

4 tablespoons salted butter

½ medium yellow onion, peeled and chopped

2 cloves garlic, peeled and finely minced

2 cups kale, chopped

5 cups chicken broth

2 cups roughly chopped cauliflower florets

2 ounces cream cheese, softened

¾ cup heavy whipping cream

¼ teaspoon xanthan gum

Per Serving

Calories: 616 | Fat: 51g | Protein: 22g | Sodium: 2,100mg | Fiber: 2g | Carbohydrates: 10g | Net Carbohydrates: 8g | Sugar: 5g

1 In a medium skillet over medium heat, brown sausage until fully cooked and no pink remains, about 15 minutes. Drain the excess fat and set sausage aside. Using the same skillet, fry bacon over medium-high heat until crispy, crumble, and set aside.

2 In a large pot over medium heat, melt butter. Add onion and sauté until onion softens and becomes translucent, about 3 minutes.

3 Add garlic and kale and sauté until kale softens, 3–5 minutes.

4 Pour broth into the pot and add cauliflower, sausage, and bacon. Increase the heat to high so the soup can come to a boil for 5 minutes, then cover and reduce the heat to a simmer over low heat. Allow the soup to simmer for 30 minutes. Remove the lid and allow it to reduce for 10 minutes, then whisk in cream cheese. Pour in heavy whipping cream, xanthan gum, and stir. Allow 2 minutes to thicken. Serve warm.

Side Dish Ideas

Soups on their own aren't always as filling as you'd like. Salads are a good option to help fill you up. You can also try a keto bread alternative such as Cheddar Bacon Biscuits (see recipe in Chapter 7).

CAJUN JAMBALAYA

If you're looking for an explosion of flavor in a one-pot dish that everyone will love, you have to try this Cajun Jambalaya. Jambalaya is a rice-based Cajun dish that originates in New Orleans, but this version swaps in cauliflower to make it keto-friendly.

Prep time 10 minutes | **Cook time** 60 minutes | **Serves 6**

2 tablespoons coconut oil

½ pound boneless, skinless chicken thigh, cubed

2¼ pounds andouille sausage links, sliced into thin rounds

½ medium yellow onion, peeled and diced

1 medium green bell pepper, seeded and diced

2 medium stalks celery, diced

2 tablespoons Cajun seasoning

5 cups chicken broth

2 tablespoons tomato paste

4 tablespoons salted butter

⅛ teaspoon dried cayenne powder

1 bay leaf

¼ teaspoon dried thyme

¼ teaspoon xanthan gum

Per Serving
Calories: 253 | Fat: 18g | Protein: 16g | Sodium: 1,589mg | Fiber: 2g | Carbohydrates: 5g | Net Carbohydrates: 3g | Sugar: 3g

1 In a large pot over medium heat, melt coconut oil. Place chicken into the pot and cook for 10 minutes or until no pink remains and internal temperature is at least 165°F.

2 Add sausage and let the fat render for 2 minutes. Add onion, bell pepper, and celery. Let the mixture cook for 3 minutes until vegetables begin to soften and become fragrant. Sprinkle with Cajun seasoning and stir for 30 seconds.

3 Pour in chicken broth, then stir in tomato paste, butter, cayenne, bay leaf, and thyme. Bring the pot to a boil for 5 minutes, then reduce and let simmer uncovered for 25 minutes, stirring occasionally. It will reduce and start to thicken. Stir in xanthan gum and let simmer for 10 more minutes, then remove from heat. Remove bay leaf. Serve warm.

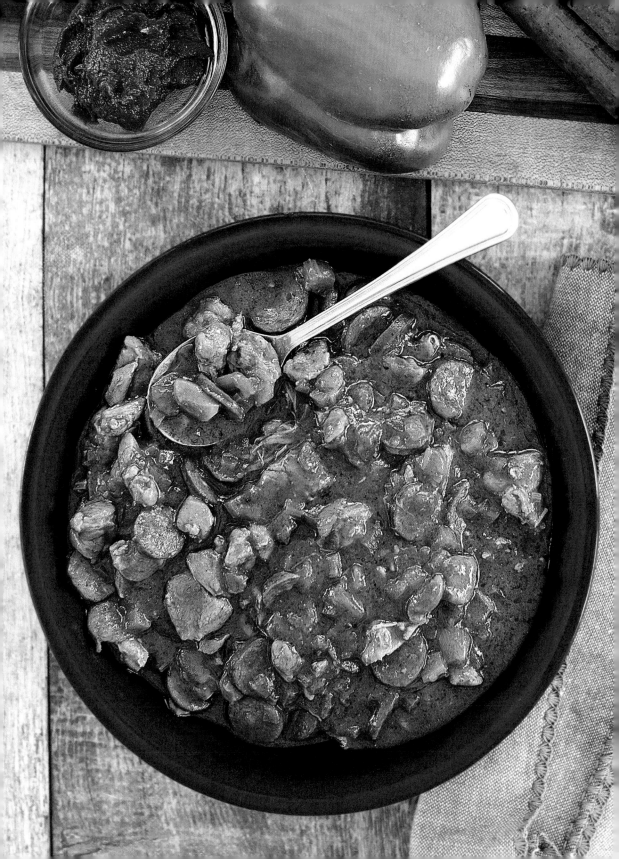

ITALIAN SAUSAGE SOUP

Shredded cabbage is an often-overlooked substitution for noodles in keto meals. Cabbage can be softer or add a little crunch depending on your preferences. It takes on the flavor of what it's cooked in, which makes it an even better swap than zucchini noodles for soup.

Prep time 10 minutes | **Cook time** 45 minutes | **Serves 4**

- **1 pound ground Italian sausage**
- **4 tablespoons salted butter**
- **¼ medium yellow onion, peeled and diced**
- **2 cloves garlic, peeled and minced**
- **5 cups chicken broth**
- **2 tablespoons tomato paste**
- **2 cups shredded green cabbage**
- **1 medium zucchini, diced**
- **2 cups spinach, chopped**

1 In a large pot over medium heat, brown sausage until no pink remains, about 12 minutes. Add butter, onion, and garlic and cook for an additional 4 minutes.

2 Pour in broth, stir in tomato paste, and then add cabbage.

3 Simmer for 20 minutes, stirring occasionally. Add zucchini and spinach and let cook for 5–7 minutes or until zucchini is tender. Serve warm.

Per Serving
Calories: 543 | Fat: 45g | Protein: 20g | Sodium: 2,159mg | Fiber: 2g | Carbohydrates: 9g | Net Carbohydrates: 7g | Sugar: 4g

SPICY PORK STEW

This dish is full of flavor and is great for leftovers! Sometimes it's hard to use up a full batch of pulled pork, so try repurposing it into this stew. This dish uses shredded cabbage as a noodle replacement and plenty of spices to give this stew a smoky and comforting taste that's perfect for cold days.

Prep time 10 minutes | **Cook time** 35 minutes | **Serves 4**

2 tablespoons salted butter

¼ medium yellow onion, peeled and finely chopped

1 large jalapeño, seeded and chopped

1 medium green bell pepper, seeded and chopped

3 cups shredded cooked pork shoulder

1 tablespoon chili powder

½ teaspoon garlic powder

2 teaspoons cumin

¼ teaspoon finely ground pink Himalayan salt

1 tablespoon tomato paste

5 cups chicken broth

2 cups shredded green cabbage

1½ cups cauliflower florets, chopped

1 In a large pot over medium heat, melt butter. Add onion and sauté 3 minutes until it begins to soften.

2 Add jalapeño and bell pepper and sauté for 4 minutes until peppers become fragrant.

3 Add pork and sprinkle in chili powder, garlic powder, cumin, and salt. Whisk tomato paste into the pot until combined, about 1 minute, then pour in broth.

4 Add cabbage and cauliflower. Simmer for 25 minutes, stirring occasionally. Serve warm.

Per Serving
Calories: 433 | Fat: 28g | Protein: 28g | Sodium: 1,477mg | Fiber: 4g | Carbohydrates: 10g | Net Carbohydrates: 6g | Sugar: 4g

Save Time

You can save time by grabbing precooked pulled pork at the store. Bulk stores often sell larger packages without any sauces that would make a great addition to this soup. Just be sure to check the label for hidden sugars.

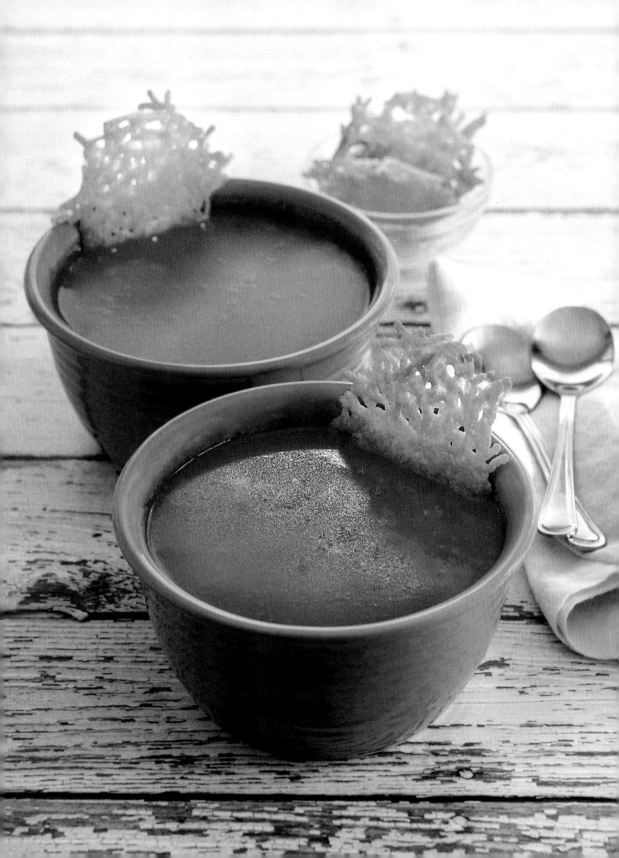

TOMATO SOUP WITH CHEESE CROUTONS

Tomato soup is a classic dish, especially as a side for grilled cheese sandwiches! This version fills the soup with cheesy, keto-friendly croutons to replicate the taste of that perfect pairing in every bite. This recipe is a bit higher in carbs than other soups in this book because it has a tomato base, but in comparison to a traditional can of tomato soup, this recipe still has much fewer carbs.

Prep time 10 minutes | **Cook time** 35 minutes | **Serves 4**

2 tablespoons salted butter

¼ medium yellow onion, peeled and diced

1 (28-ounce) can crushed tomatoes

⅛ teaspoon garlic powder

⅛ teaspoon finely ground pink Himalayan salt

⅛ teaspoon ground black pepper

3 cups vegetable broth

½ cup heavy whipping cream

1 cup shredded Parmesan

Per Serving
Calories: 313 | Fat: 22g | Protein: 12g | Sodium: 1,218mg | Fiber: 5g | Carbohydrates: 19g | Net Carbohydrates: 14g | Sugar: 11g

1 In a large pot over medium heat, melt butter. Add onion and sauté for 3 minutes until it begins to soften.

2 Add tomatoes, garlic powder, salt, pepper, and broth. Bring to a boil, then simmer for 20 minutes. Pour the mixture into a blender and purée. Pour the soup back into the pot and pour in heavy whipping cream and remove from heat.

3 Preheat the oven to 400°F. Line a baking sheet with parchment paper.

4 Form 1-tablespoon mounds of cheese and place at least 2" apart on the prepared baking sheet. Bake for 7–10 minutes or until golden and crispy. Let cool for 10 minutes.

5 Immediately before serving the soup, top with the baked cheese.

Make It a Meal

Craving more grilled cheese goodness? Use the quick bread recipe from the 90-Second Bread Tuna Melt (see recipe in Chapter 6) to sop up the end of this savory soup!

TACO SOUP

Everything you love about Taco Tuesday is coming to a hot and creamy bowl near you! This flavorful soup is filled with all of your favorite taco tastes and the perfect kick to wake up your taste buds. The protein helps make this a filling meal. Feel free to add your favorite toppings such as shredded cheese or a spoonful of sour cream. Or add crushed cheese crisps for a big crunch in each bite.

Prep time 10 minutes | **Cook time** 45 minutes | **Serves 6**

½ tablespoon chili powder

1 teaspoon cumin

½ teaspoon garlic powder

⅛ teaspoon ground black pepper

⅛ teaspoon finely ground sea salt

1 pound boneless, skinless chicken thigh

2 tablespoons coconut oil

¼ cup chopped peeled white onion

½ medium green bell pepper, seeded and chopped

1 (14.5-ounce) can diced tomatoes, drained

5 cups chicken broth

2 tablespoons tomato paste

2 tablespoons salted butter

¼ cup chopped fresh cilantro

1 In a small bowl, mix chili powder, cumin, garlic powder, black pepper, and salt. Sprinkle the mixture on both sides of each chicken thigh.

2 In a medium pot over medium heat, melt coconut oil. Place chicken into the pot and cook for 12 minutes or until fully cooked and internal temperature reaches at least 165°F. Set chicken aside on a cutting board.

3 Add onion and bell pepper to the pot and sauté 3 minutes until vegetables begin to soften. Add diced tomatoes and pour in chicken broth. Whisk in tomato paste.

4 Chop chicken into bite-sized pieces and add to the pot. Bring to a boil for 5 minutes, then reduce the heat to low and simmer for 25 minutes. The liquid in the soup should reduce by about 1 cup.

5 Turn off the heat and add butter. Stir until fully melted. To serve, garnish with cilantro.

Per Serving
Calories: 175 | Fat: 9g | Protein: 13g | Sodium: 1,008mg | Fiber: 2g | Carbohydrates: 7g | Net Carbohydrates: 5g | Sugar: 4g

NOODLELESS LASAGNA SOUP

This soup is the best way to enjoy all the comforting flavors of lasagna with minimal prep. If you don't think you like ricotta, this recipe might just change your mind—it makes all the difference in this soup, adding a rich creaminess. Pair this soup with a crisp salad or Easy Cheese Bread in Chapter 7.

Prep time 15 minutes | **Cook time** 40 minutes | **Serves 4**

1 pound 80/20 ground beef

2 tablespoons salted butter

¼ medium yellow onion, peeled and diced

2 tablespoons tomato paste

½ teaspoon dried basil

½ teaspoon garlic powder

½ teaspoon finely ground pink Himalayan salt

¼ teaspoon ground black pepper

¼ teaspoon dried oregano

1 (14-ounce) can diced tomatoes, drained

3½ cups beef broth

½ cup ricotta

½ cup shredded mozzarella

½ cup grated Parmesan

2 tablespoons chopped fresh parsley

1 In a medium pot over medium heat, brown ground beef until no pink remains, about 10 minutes. Drain the excess grease, then return the pot to the heat.

2 Melt the butter in the pan. Sauté onion for 3 minutes until it begins to soften. Whisk in tomato paste, then sprinkle in basil, garlic powder, salt, pepper, and oregano. Let cook for 1 minute.

3 Pour in diced tomatoes and broth. Let simmer uncovered for 25 minutes.

4 In a small bowl, mix ricotta, mozzarella, and Parmesan. To serve soup, spoon the cheese mixture over each bowl of soup. Garnish with parsley.

Per Serving

Calories: 421 | Fat: 24g | Protein: 30g | Sodium: 912mg | Fiber: 2g | Carbohydrates: 12g | Net Carbohydrates: 10g | Sugar: 5g

Freeze It!

This recipe makes an excellent freezer meal. Simply omit the cheeses until you're ready to enjoy. Place the soup into a freezer bag and store up to 3 months for best freshness. Let it thaw in cool water, then reheat in the microwave or on the stovetop. Top with fresh cheese before serving.

CHICKEN AND DUMPLING SOUP

This flavorful soup always has people asking for seconds! The cheesy dumplings don't taste the same as traditional dumplings, because the ingredients are very different, but they are delicious nonetheless—and they won't make you go over your carb limit for the day.

Prep time 10 minutes | **Cook time** 40 minutes | **Serves 4**

2 tablespoons salted butter

¼ medium white onion, peeled and chopped

1 large carrot, peeled and finely chopped

2 medium stalks celery, chopped

1 clove garlic, peeled and finely minced

¼ teaspoon dried oregano

1 bay leaf

2 cups shredded cooked chicken thigh

5 cups chicken broth

½ cup heavy whipping cream

½ cup shredded mozzarella

1 tablespoon unsalted butter

½ cup finely ground blanched almond flour

¼ teaspoon baking soda

¼ teaspoon white vinegar

Per Serving
Calories: 467 | Fat: 33g | Protein: 28g | Sodium: 1,446mg | Fiber: 2g | Carbohydrates: 11g | Net Carbohydrates: 9g | Sugar: 5g

1 In a large pot over medium heat, melt salted butter. Add onion, carrot, and celery, then sauté for 5 minutes until fragrant and beginning to soften.

2 Add garlic, oregano, bay leaf, and chicken, then pour in broth. Simmer uncovered over low heat for 25 minutes. Pour in the heavy cream.

3 In a large microwave-safe bowl, mix mozzarella, unsalted butter, and almond flour. Microwave for 45 seconds, then stir until a soft ball of dough forms. Stir in baking soda and vinegar.

4 Separate the dough into 2-tablespoon heaps and place on top of the soup. Cover and let cook for 5 minutes. Remove bay leaf from the soup. Let cool for 10 minutes. Serve warm.

BROCCOLI CHEDDAR SOUP

You'll love the keto-friendly spin on this popular restaurant favorite even more than the original! The cauliflower makes the soup thick without the use of xanthan gum or other thickeners, and it adds more depth of flavor. This soup is sure to be a family favorite.

Prep time 10 minutes | **Cook time** 30 minutes | **Serves 4**

2 tablespoons salted butter
¼ medium yellow onion, peeled and chopped
1 clove garlic, peeled and finely minced
5 cups chicken broth
1 (12-ounce) bag riced cauliflower
1 cup broccoli, chopped
¼ cup shredded peeled carrot
2 ounces cream cheese, softened
¾ cup heavy whipping cream
6 ounces sharp Cheddar, grated
4 slices bacon, cooked and crumbled

Per Serving
Calories: 531 | Fat: 42g | Protein: 21g | Sodium: 1,767mg | Fiber: 3g | Carbohydrates: 11g | Net Carbohydrates: 8g | Sugar: 6g

1 In a large pot over medium heat, melt butter. Sauté onion for 3 minutes or until it begins to soften. Add garlic and sauté for an additional 30 seconds.

2 Pour in broth and cauliflower. Bring to a boil for 5 minutes. Carefully pour the soup into a blender and purée until all cauliflower is broken down and smooth. Carefully pour the soup back into the pot on the stove.

3 Add broccoli and carrot to the soup. Simmer uncovered for 20 minutes to reduce.

4 In a small bowl, mix cream cheese and heavy whipping cream. Scoop the mixture into the pot and stir until combined.

5 Whisk in Cheddar until the soup is completely smooth, about 1 minute. Garnish with crumbled bacon. Serve warm.

CHICKEN ZOODLE SOUP

This recipe will be an instant classic in your kitchen because the low-carb ingredients in it, including the spiralized zucchini that mimics the noodles, more than make up for the carb-heavy noodles in the original. This recipe has all the classic ingredients—yes, even the carrots. Though some choose to avoid carrots on a strict ketogenic diet, they can be enjoyed in moderation.

Prep time 10 minutes | **Cook time** 50 minutes | **Serves 4**

2 tablespoons coconut oil

1½ pounds boneless, skinless chicken thigh, cubed

4 tablespoons salted butter

½ medium white onion, peeled and diced

2 cloves garlic, peeled and finely minced

2 medium stalks celery, chopped

1 medium carrot, peeled and sliced

6 cups chicken broth

2 teaspoons apple cider vinegar

1 bay leaf

¼ teaspoon dried oregano

¼ teaspoon ground black pepper

⅛ teaspoon sea salt

4 medium zucchini, spiralized

Per Serving
Calories: 439 | Fat: 24g | Protein: 39g | Sodium: 1,729mg | Fiber: 3g | Carbohydrates: 12g | Net Carbohydrates: 9g | Sugar: 8g

1 In a large pot over medium heat, melt coconut oil. Sear chicken on each side, then stir and continue cooking until no pink remains, about 10 minutes.

2 Melt butter in the pot, then add onion and sauté 3 minutes until it begins to soften. Add garlic and sauté for 30 seconds.

3 Add celery and carrot and continue to cook for 3 minutes, stirring occasionally.

4 Pour in broth and vinegar, then add bay leaf, oregano, pepper, and salt. Bring to a boil over medium heat, then let simmer uncovered for 30 minutes.

5 Remove bay leaf, then add zucchini. Turn off the heat and cover for 5 minutes to allow the zucchini to cook from residual heat. This will prevent soggy zoodles. Serve warm.

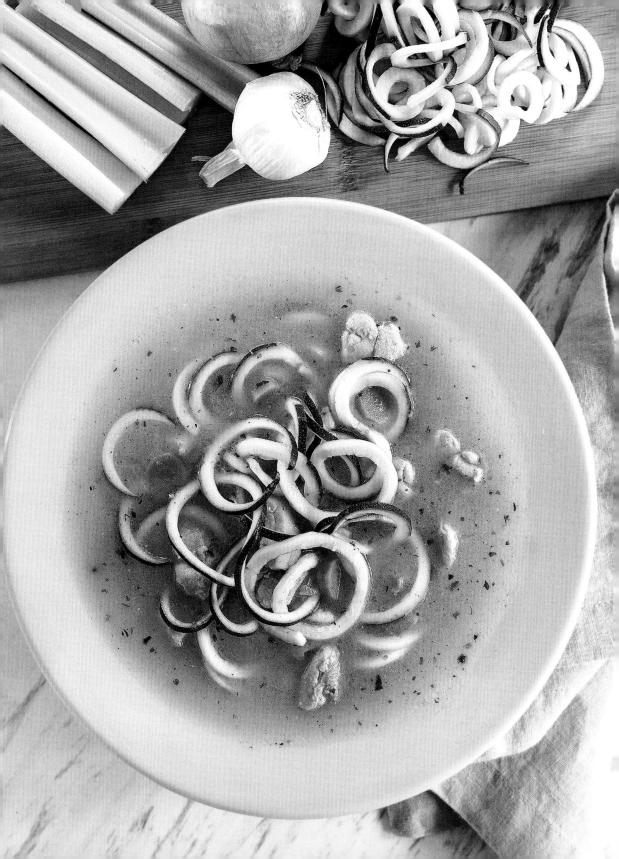

REUBEN SOUP

Reubens are such delicious and filling sandwiches, but the bread is loaded with enough carbs to kick you out of ketosis. As a tasty, creamy soup, it offers all the tangy flavor and warm comfort with a fraction of the carbs! If you don't like the strong taste of Swiss cheese, you can always substitute Monterey jack.

Prep time 10 minutes | **Cook time** 25 minutes | **Serves 4**

4 tablespoons salted butter

¼ medium yellow onion, peeled and finely diced

1 clove garlic, peeled and finely minced

4 cups chicken broth

12 ounces frozen cauliflower, chopped

½ pound cooked corned beef, chopped

1 cup sauerkraut

2 ounces cream cheese

½ cup heavy whipping cream

1 cup shredded Swiss cheese

Per Serving
Calories: 542 | Fat: 42g | Protein: 29g | Sodium: 1,903mg | Fiber: 3g | Carbohydrates: 11g | Net Carbohydrates: 8g | Sugar: 6g

1 In a large pot over medium heat, melt butter. Add onion and sauté 3 minutes until it begins to soften. Add garlic and sauté for 30 seconds, then pour in broth and add cauliflower.

2 Add beef and sauerkraut to the pot. Let simmer for 20 minutes, stirring occasionally. In a small bowl, whisk cream cheese and heavy whipping cream. Whisk the mixture into the soup until smooth, then add Swiss cheese, stirring until melted and creamy, about 1 minute. Serve warm.

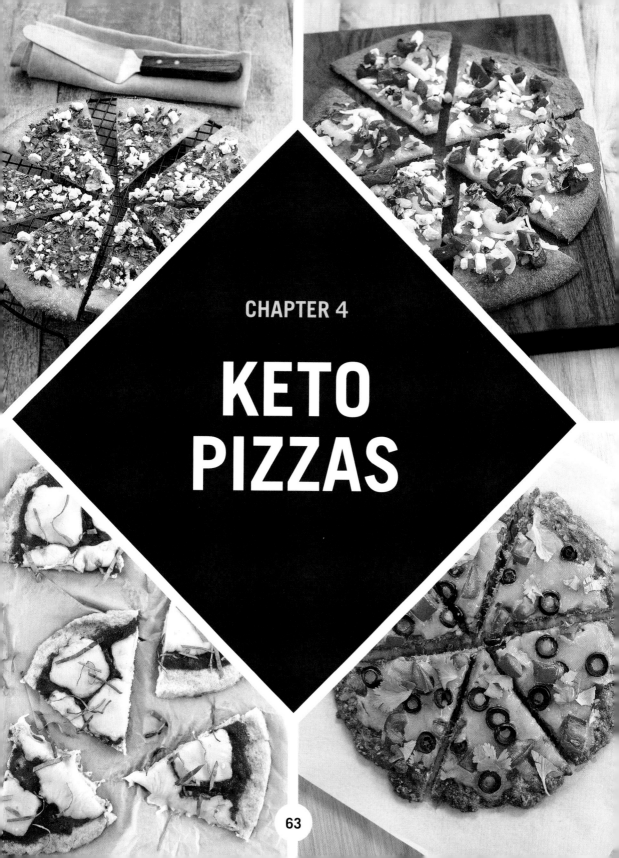

CHAPTER 4

KETO PIZZAS

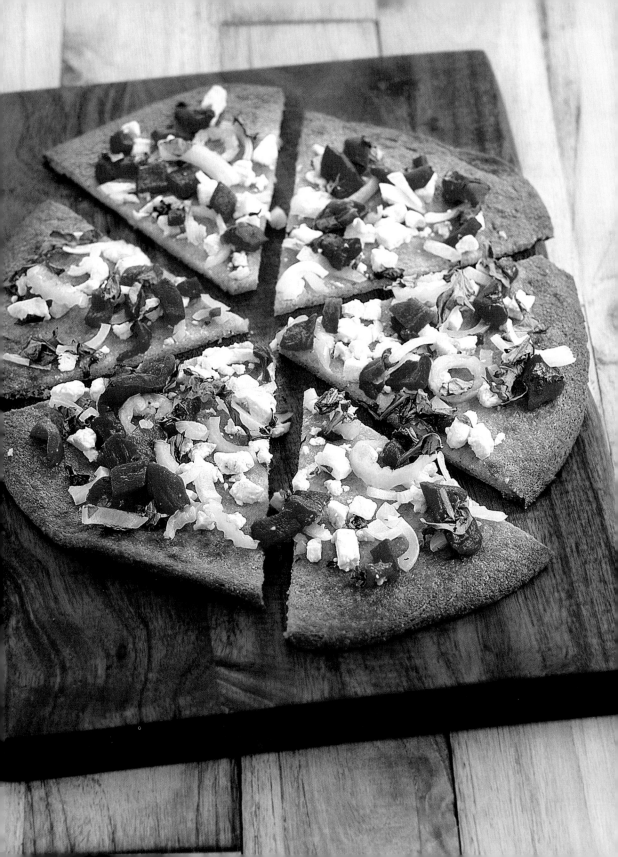

MEDITERRA-NEAN VEGETABLE PIZZA

This pizza satisfies the keto diet's emphasis on vegetables. This loaded pizza is packed with micronutrients and satisfying flavor in every bite. It's like a pizza and a salad all in one!

Prep time 10 minutes | **Cook time** 25 minutes | **Serves 6**

1 cup finely ground blanched almond flour
2½ cups shredded mozzarella
2 ounces cream cheese
2 ounces crumbled feta
10 banana pepper rings
¼ medium yellow onion, peeled and sliced
2 roasted red peppers, chopped
½ cup spinach, chopped

Per Serving
Calories: 312 | Fat: 22g | Protein: 20g | Sodium: 376mg | Fiber: 3g | Carbohydrates: 12g | Net Carbohydrates: 9g | Sugar: 4g

1 Preheat the oven to 400°F. Line a baking sheet with parchment paper.

2 In a large microwave-safe bowl, gently mix almond flour, mozzarella, and cream cheese. Microwave for 30 seconds, stir, and microwave an additional 30 seconds until the mixture is melted. Stir until a soft ball of dough forms.

3 Wet your hands with a little water to prevent the dough from sticking. Press the dough out on the prepared baking sheet into a 12" round.

4 Bake for 5 minutes. Remove it from the oven and top with feta, pepper rings, onion, red peppers, and spinach. Place back into the oven for an additional 15 minutes to finish cooking the crust and warm the vegetables. Let cool for 10 minutes before serving. Serve warm.

Balancing Your Macros

This recipe has more vegetables and carbs than some other meals. Some people choose to be as close to 0 carbs as possible, while others enjoy carb limits of 20 grams per day (or sometimes even up to 50 grams per day). Plan your meals ahead of time so you can offset one higher-carb meal with lower-carb options the rest of the day.

5-MINUTE SKILLET PIZZA

While many keto pizza alternatives are delicious, they usually require more time than traditional pizzas. This 5-Minute Skillet Pizza is great when you don't have time for a large meal. The cheese crisps up like a thin-crust pizza to give you a big crunch while delivering all the flavors you've been craving.

Prep time 1 minute | **Cook time** 5 minutes | **Serves 1**

1 cup shredded mozzarella

2 tablespoons low-carb marinara sauce

7 slices pepperoni

Per Serving
Calories: 401 | Fat: 29g | Protein: 32g | Sodium: 926mg | Fiber: 1g | Carbohydrates: 7g | Net Carbohydrates: 6g | Sugar: 2g

1 In a medium skillet over medium heat, sprinkle cheese in a circle to cover the bottom of the pan. Let cheese melt for 30 seconds, then spoon marinara sauce over cheese and place pepperoni on top.

2 Continue to cook for 3–4 minutes until the cheese is golden and crispy on the bottom. Let cool for 2 minutes before serving.

Pan Quality

Be sure to use a good-quality nonstick pan without scratches for this recipe. That will eliminate the need to grease it up beforehand and will keep your yummy pizza intact when you take it out of the skillet!

CRUSTLESS SUPREME PIZZA

This pizza is so full of gooey, meaty, and cheesy goodness that you'll forget it doesn't even have a crust! Crustless pizzas are popular on the keto diet because they're very simple, and the carbs you save by ditching the crust can be used to really bulk up the yummy toppings! This recipe includes some higher-carb vegetables like onions and olives that you might not necessarily indulge in every day.

Prep time 10 minutes | **Cook time** 25 minutes | **Serves 6**

1 pound ground sausage
1 cup low-carb pizza sauce
14 slices pepperoni
1 cup shredded mozzarella
½ medium green bell pepper, seeded and chopped
¼ medium white onion, peeled and sliced
¼ cup sliced black olives
¼ cup grated Parmesan

Per Serving
Calories: 365 | Fat: 27g | Protein: 21g | Sodium: 522mg | Fiber: 1g | Carbohydrates: 7g | Net Carbohydrates: 6g | Sugar: 2g

1 Preheat the oven to 425°F.

2 In a 12" cast-iron skillet (or other oven-safe skillet) over medium heat, brown sausage until no pink remains, about 10 minutes.

3 Drain the excess grease from the pan and pour pizza sauce into the pan. Place pepperoni around the pan and sprinkle mozzarella evenly on top.

4 Add bell pepper, onion, and olives on top of cheese. Place the cast-iron skillet into the oven and bake for 15 minutes or until the cheese is brown and bubbling. Sprinkle with grated Parmesan and let cool for 5–10 minutes before serving. To serve, use a large spoon to separate into six portions and scoop onto plates.

MEAT LOVER'S CALZONE

A calzone is essentially a savory turnover made of pizza dough and filled with pizza toppings. This version perfectly replicates the bready texture of the original and stuffs each calzone full of delicious protein to keep you full. It's like a cheat meal with no guilt!

Prep time 15 minutes | **Cook time** 25 minutes | **Serves 4**

1½ cups finely ground blanched almond flour

2½ cups shredded mozzarella

2 ounces cream cheese

1 teaspoon baking powder

½ teaspoon apple cider vinegar

14 slices pepperoni

½ cup diced cooked ham

4 slices cooked bacon, crumbled

2 tablespoons salted butter, melted

1 clove garlic, peeled and minced

2 tablespoons finely chopped fresh parsley

2 tablespoons grated Parmesan

1 cup low-carb marinara sauce

1 Preheat the oven to 400°F. Line a baking sheet with parchment paper.

2 In a large microwave-safe bowl, mix almond flour, mozzarella, and cream cheese. Microwave for 45 seconds, then stir. Microwave for an additional 15 seconds, then add baking powder and vinegar. Stir until a soft ball of dough forms.

3 Press the dough out on the prepared baking sheet to a 12" round. Place pepperoni, ham, and bacon on half of the round. Fold the other half of the dough over the toppings and press the edges to seal, rolling them gently, if necessary.

4 In a small bowl, whisk butter and garlic. Brush the mixture gently over the calzone. Bake for 20 minutes until golden.

5 Sprinkle parsley and Parmesan over top. Let cool for 10 minutes before serving with marinara sauce for dipping.

Per Serving

Calories: 746 | Fat: 56g | Protein: 38g | Sodium: 1,515mg | Fiber: 5g | Carbohydrates: 17g | Net Carbohydrates: 12g | Sugar: 6g

Preventing Sticking

When working with cheese-based dough, wetting your hands with a little water can help prevent sticking. It won't affect the integrity of the dough, but it will help you press it out evenly without the dough getting too stuck to your fingers.

BACON CHEESE- BURGER PIZZA

Have you ever struggled to choose between burgers and pizza for dinner? This amazing recipe marries the two in a unique and flavorful combination. It's just like your favorite fast-food burger on a crispy, low-carb crust, with a tangy sauce to bring it all together. Don't forget the pickles!

Prep time 15 minutes | **Cook time** 40 minutes | **Serves 6**

¼ pound 80/20 ground beef
⅛ teaspoon pink Himalayan salt
⅛ teaspoon ground black pepper
4 slices bacon
2 cups shredded mozzarella
½ cup grated Parmesan
2 large eggs
¼ cup shredded Cheddar
10 slices dill pickles, diced
2 tablespoons mayonnaise
2 teaspoons low-carb ketchup
1 teaspoon soy sauce
2 tablespoons peeled and finely diced yellow onion

Per Serving
Calories: 287 | Fat: 21g | Protein: 21g | Sodium: 769mg | Fiber: 0g | Carbohydrates: 4g | Net Carbohydrates: 4g | Sugar: 0g

1 Preheat the oven to 400°F. Line a large baking sheet with parchment paper.

2 In a medium skillet over medium heat, brown ground beef until no pink remains, about 10 minutes. Drain the excess fat and sprinkle beef with salt and pepper. Place beef in a small dish and set aside. Cook bacon in the same skillet over medium heat until browned and crispy, about 10 minutes. Set aside on paper towels to absorb fat. Crumble bacon.

3 In a large bowl, mix mozzarella, Parmesan, and eggs until the entire mixture is coated in eggs; it will be wet but not overly runny.

4 Use a rubber spatula to scoop the mixture into the center of the prepared baking sheet. Press out into a 12" circle.

5 Scatter ground beef around the cheese mixture and sprinkle with Cheddar. Top with pickles and bake for 15 minutes. Carefully pull out the rack and add crumbled bacon. Return to the oven to finish cooking for an additional 5 minutes. The cheese crust should be firm and golden brown when done. Let cool for 10 minutes, then slice into six pieces.

6 In a small bowl, mix mayonnaise, ketchup, soy sauce, and onion. Feel free to add ½ teaspoon water to thin out the mixture if it seems too thick. Drizzle over pizza or reserve for dipping.

CAULIFLOWER CRUST MARGHERITA PIZZA

Cauliflower continues to show its extreme versatility in this recipe. The crust is low carb, and the cauliflower taste is very unnoticeable. You'll feel good about feeding your family this nutrient-packed pizza. If you want to shake things up a bit, drizzle some balsamic vinaigrette on top of the pizza after it comes out of the oven!

Prep time 10 minutes | **Cook time** 25 minutes | **Serves 6**

2 (12-ounce) steamer bags cauliflower florets

1 large egg

½ cup shredded mozzarella

¼ cup grated Parmesan

½ cup low-carb marinara sauce

6 ounces fresh mozzarella, thinly sliced

4 leaves fresh basil, thinly sliced

Per Serving

Calories: 162 | Fat: 9g | Protein: 12g | Sodium: 303mg | Fiber: 3g | Carbohydrates: 8g | Net Carbohydrates: 5g | Sugar: 4g

1 Preheat the oven to 400°F. Line a large baking sheet with parchment paper.

2 Cook the steamer bags of cauliflower according to package instructions. Allow to cool and then use a kitchen towel or cheesecloth to remove as much excess moisture as possible. Then place cauliflower into a food processor. Add egg, mozzarella, and Parmesan and pulse for 20 seconds until egg is fully incorporated.

3 Scoop the mixture onto the prepared baking sheet. Wet your hands with water to prevent sticking, then press the mixture into a 12" round.

4 Bake the crust for 10 minutes. Remove and add marinara sauce and mozzarella. Return to the oven for an additional 10 minutes or until mozzarella is melted.

5 Allow the pizza to cool for 10 minutes before serving. Sprinkle basil on top of the pizza, then slice into six pieces. Serve warm.

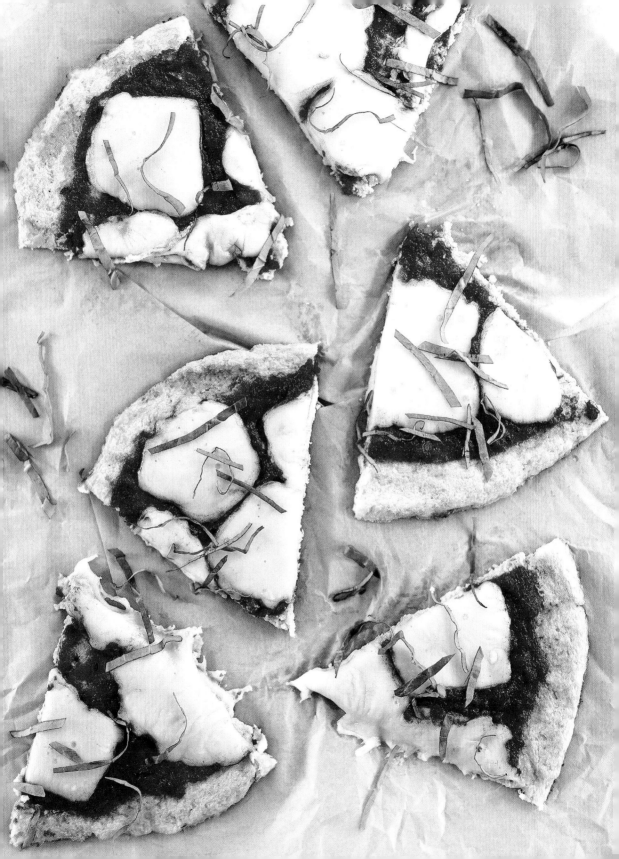

BUFFALO CHICKEN CRUST PIZZA

If you're a lover of all things spicy, this protein-packed pizza is for you! By using chicken as the crust, you eliminate all the carbs that a normal pizza crust would have, plus you get even more succulent flavor in every single bite!

Prep time 10 minutes | **Cook time** 35 minutes | **Serves 6**

1 pound ground chicken thigh
1 cup shredded mozzarella
⅓ cup buffalo sauce
¼ teaspoon garlic powder
⅛ teaspoon ground black pepper
1 cup shredded mild Cheddar
6 tablespoons ranch dressing
¼ cup crumbled blue cheese

Per Serving
Calories: 320 | Fat: 23g | Protein: 24g | Sodium: 874mg | Fiber: 0g | Carbohydrates: 2g | Net Carbohydrates: 2g | Sugar: 1g

1 Preheat the oven to 400°F. Line a large baking sheet with parchment paper.

2 In a large bowl, mix chicken, mozzarella, buffalo sauce, garlic powder, and pepper.

3 Press the chicken mixture into a 14" round shape on the prepared baking sheet. Bake for 20 minutes.

4 Remove and sprinkle with Cheddar. Return to the oven for an additional 15 minutes or until internal temperature is 165°F. Chicken will be browned around the edges and cheese will be golden.

5 Drizzle with ranch dressing and sprinkle with blue cheese. Let cool for 10 minutes before serving.

PEPPERONI PIZZA

The crust on this pizza is a mixture of cheeses that crisps up golden brown when cooked and is similar to a thin-crust pizza. It doesn't rise like pizza, but you won't even miss the bready texture once you're enjoying all the flavor of this Friday night classic.

Prep time 10 minutes | **Cook time** 25 minutes | **Serves 6**

1 cup finely ground blanched almond flour
¼ teaspoon dried basil
⅛ teaspoon dried oregano
⅛ teaspoon garlic powder
2½ cups shredded mozzarella
2 ounces cream cheese, softened
1 large egg
½ cup low-carb pizza sauce
¾ cup shredded mild Cheddar
14 slices pepperoni

Per Serving
Calories: 379 | Fat: 27g | Protein: 23g | Sodium: 552mg | Fiber: 2g | Carbohydrates: 11g | Net Carbohydrates: 9g | Sugar: 2g

1 Preheat the oven to 400°F. Line a large baking sheet with parchment paper.

2 In a large microwave-safe bowl, mix almond flour, basil, oregano, garlic powder, mozzarella, and cream cheese. Microwave for 45 seconds, then stir. Microwave an additional 15 seconds, then stir until a smooth ball forms.

3 Crack egg open into the bowl and fold into the soft dough, using your hands as necessary. Wet your hands with a little water to prevent sticking as needed.

4 On the prepared baking sheet, press the dough into a 14" round. Bake for 5 minutes.

5 Remove from the oven and pour pizza sauce onto the crust. Top with Cheddar and pepperoni, then return to the oven to bake for an additional 15 minutes or until cheese is melted and browned. Let cool for 10 minutes before serving.

Sauce Swaps

Red sauce is the traditional choice for pizza sauce, but ranch can be great too! Try using ¼ cup ranch dressing or alfredo sauce in place of the red sauce.

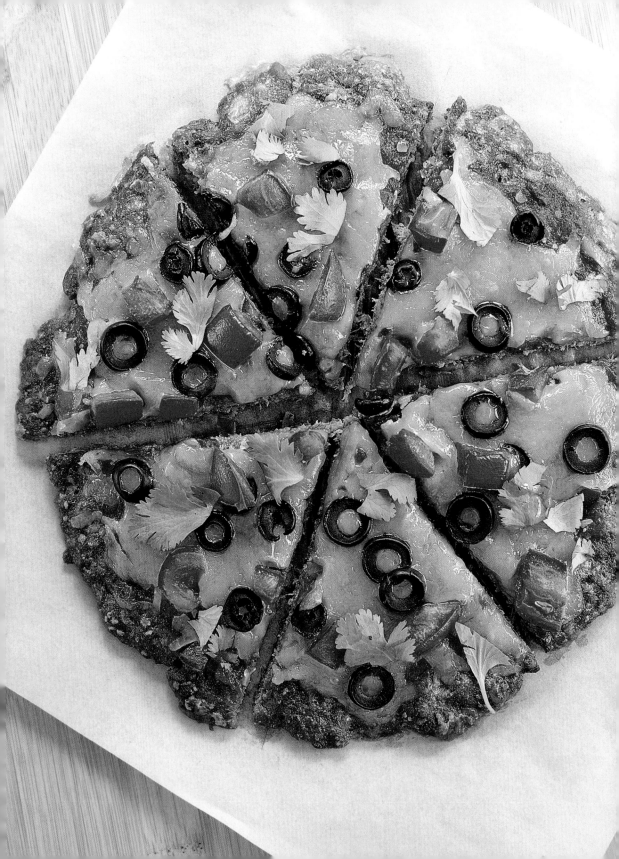

CHICKEN CRUST TACO PIZZA

This recipe uses chicken as the crust for edge-to-edge, deliciously seasoned taco flavor in every bite. Plus, it's piled high with all of your favorite toppings, making it a filling meal your whole family will devour!

Prep time 10 minutes | **Cook time** 35 minutes | **Serves 6**

1 pound ground chicken thigh
½ cup grated Parmesan
½ cup shredded mozzarella
1 tablespoon chili powder
2 teaspoons ground cumin
1 teaspoon ground paprika
¼ teaspoon ground black pepper
¼ teaspoon garlic powder
½ cup salsa
¾ cup shredded mild Cheddar
⅛ cup sliced black olives
½ Roma tomato, seeded and chopped
2 tablespoons chopped fresh cilantro

1 Preheat the oven to 375°F. Line a large baking sheet with parchment paper.

2 In a large bowl, mix chicken, Parmesan, mozzarella, chili powder, cumin, paprika, pepper, and garlic powder.

3 Wet your hands to prevent sticking, and press the ground chicken mixture out into a 14" round. Bake for 20 minutes.

4 Remove the pan and pour salsa over the chicken crust. Top with Cheddar, olives, and tomato, then continue to bake for an additional 15 minutes or until cheese is bubbling and brown and the crust is fully cooked to at least 165°F internal temperature.

5 Garnish with cilantro and let cool for 10 minutes before serving. Feel free to add your favorite taco toppings or dip in sour cream. Serve warm.

Per Serving
Calories: 246 | Fat: 15g | Protein: 22g | Sodium: 551mg | Fiber: 1g | Carbohydrates: 5g | Net Carbohydrates: 4g | Sugar: 2g

Freeze It!

Chicken crust is great for freezing for later use. For easy dinners, just make a big batch, separate the dough into mini pizzas, place between parchment paper, and store in a sealed zippered freezer bag in the freezer for up to 3 months for best freshness. Defrost in the microwave, then top and bake for 15 minutes.

CHICKEN BACON RANCH PIZZA

This is a family favorite that even the pickiest eaters may enjoy! Though this crust doesn't resemble bread, it has far more flavor than a flour-based dough, not to mention a good dose of protein. This crust is sturdy enough that you can even hold it like a real slice of pizza. For an extra crunch, crisp up the crust in a skillet after cooking or when reheating leftovers.

Prep time 10 minutes | **Cook time** 35 minutes | **Serves 6**

1 pound ground chicken thigh
½ cup shredded mozzarella
½ (1-ounce) packet dry ranch seasoning
1 cup shredded sharp Cheddar
6 slices bacon, cooked and crumbled
¼ cup ranch dressing

Per Serving
Calories: 276 | Fat: 17g | Protein: 24g | Sodium: 598mg | Fiber: 0g | Carbohydrates: 2g | Net Carbohydrates: 2g | Sugar: 0g

1 Preheat the oven to 375°F. Line a large baking sheet with parchment paper.

2 In a large bowl, mix chicken, mozzarella, and ranch seasoning.

3 On the prepared baking sheet, press the ground chicken mixture into a 10" × 12" rectangle. Bake for 15 minutes, then remove from the oven and top with Cheddar and bacon.

4 Return to the oven and bake for an additional 20 minutes or until chicken is cooked through to 165°F and the cheese is melted and browned. Drizzle with ranch dressing to serve.

Make It Mini

To make a fun, hands-on family dinner, split this recipe into four smaller pizzas so everyone can decide how they want to top theirs! Add everyone's favorite vegetables and even more sauce choices to the table and let everyone get creative.

PHILLY CHEESESTEAK PIZZA

Shredded cheese is delicious on a pizza, but with cheese sauce it's even tastier! This Monterey jack cheese sauce is easy to make and tastes delicious with the crispy pieces of steak and green bell peppers. The buttery crust will have you forgetting all about bread. For an extra burst of flavor, add ¼ cup jalapeño juice to the steak while it's cooking!

Prep time 10 minutes | **Cook time** 35 minutes | **Serves 6**

1½ cups shredded mozzarella

¾ cup finely ground blanched almond flour

3 ounces cream cheese, divided

1 pound shaved sirloin steak

⅛ teaspoon finely ground pink Himalayan salt

⅛ teaspoon ground black pepper

2 tablespoons salted butter

¼ medium white onion, peeled and chopped

¼ cup heavy whipping cream

¾ cup shredded Monterey jack

½ medium green bell pepper, seeded and diced

Per Serving
Calories: 488 | Fat: 34g | Protein: 32g | Sodium: 385mg | Fiber: 1g | Carbohydrates: 8g | Net Carbohydrates: 7g | Sugar: 2g

1 Preheat the oven to 400°F. Line a large baking sheet with parchment paper.

2 In a large microwave-safe bowl, mix mozzarella, almond flour, and 2 ounces cream cheese. Microwave for 45 seconds, then stir. Microwave for an additional 15 seconds, then stir into a smooth ball.

3 Place the dough onto the prepared baking sheet and form a 12" round.

4 In a medium skillet over medium heat, cook steak. Sprinkle with salt and black pepper and continue cooking until no pink remains, about 12 minutes. Remove steak from the pan and set aside.

5 Return the skillet to medium heat and melt butter. Add onion and sauté for 3 minutes until soft. Whisk in the remaining cream cheese and heavy whipping cream until smooth, about 30 seconds. Sprinkle in Monterey jack and whisk until smooth and the cheese mixture thickens, about 1 minute.

6 Spread the cheese sauce over the uncooked crust and sprinkle with steak and green bell pepper. Bake for 15 minutes or until edges are golden. Let cool for 10 minutes. Serve warm.

SPINACH AND FETA PIZZA

You'll be amazed at how creamy the crust of this pizza tastes— yes, the crust! It's crispy on the outside and creamy on the inside, which eliminates the need for any more sauces besides a drizzle of oil. The toppings are light and make this a great choice for lunch or even as an appetizer (cut into sticks). Don't let the size fool you; this recipe is high in fat and even one slice will keep you full! Feel free to top with a sprinkle of crushed red pepper for a spicy kick.

Prep time 5 minutes | **Cook time** 20 minutes | **Serves 6**

1 cup finely ground blanched almond flour
2½ cups shredded mozzarella
2 ounces cream cheese
2 tablespoons olive oil
1½ cups chopped baby spinach
½ cup crumbled feta

Per Serving
Calories: 346 | Fat: 26g | Protein: 20g | Sodium: 404mg | Fiber: 2g | Carbohydrates: 10g | Net Carbohydrates: 8g | Sugar: 2g

1 Preheat the oven to 400°F. Line a large baking sheet with parchment paper.

2 In a large microwave-safe bowl, mix almond flour, mozzarella, and cream cheese. Microwave for 45 seconds, stir, place back in for an additional 15 seconds, and then stir until a soft ball of dough forms.

3 On the prepared baking sheet, press the dough into a 12" round. Wet your hands with a little water to help prevent sticking while you press out the dough.

4 Drizzle olive oil over the crust and top with spinach and feta. Bake for 17 minutes or until edges are browned. Let cool for 10 minutes before serving.

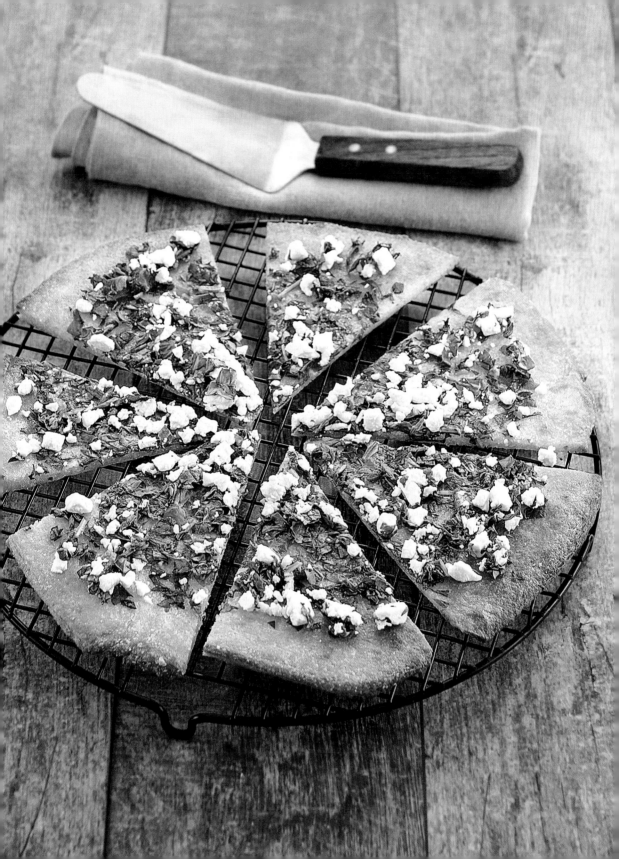

EASY SAUSAGE CRUST BREAKFAST PIZZA

Mornings just got more delicious! This pizza has a crust made out of sausage for maximum breakfast flavor. Topped with a delicious gravy made from the excess grease and fluffy eggs, this is the perfect Saturday breakfast to get your day going.

Prep time 10 minutes | **Cook time** 40 minutes | **Serves 6**

1 pound pork breakfast sausage
2 tablespoons salted butter
6 large eggs
½ cup heavy whipping cream
¼ teaspoon finely ground pink Himalayan salt
⅛ teaspoon ground black pepper
1 cup shredded sharp Cheddar
4 tablespoons sour cream
½ cup salsa

Per Serving
Calories: 478 | Fat: 37g
Protein: 23g | Sodium: 1,181mg |
Fiber: 1g | Carbohydrates: 5g | Net
Carbohydrates: 4g | Sugar: 3g

1 Preheat the oven to 400°F. Line a 12" round cake pan with parchment paper.

2 Press out the breakfast sausage to cover the bottom of the prepared pan and come slightly up the sides. Bake for 20 minutes.

3 In a medium skillet over medium heat, melt butter, then crack open eggs into the pan, then pour in the heavy whipping cream. Whisk in salt and pepper and continue cooking for 5 minutes or until eggs are softly scrambled.

4 Remove the sausage crust from the oven and add the egg mixture and top with Cheddar. Bake for an additional 15 minutes or until cheese is melted and sausage is completely cooked through and no pink remains. Let cool for 10 minutes before slicing. Serve warm alongside sour cream and salsa.

Prep It Ahead

Busy mornings? You can prepare this pizza the night before to make breakfast a breeze! Just make this the night before, then warm for a minute in the microwave when you're ready to eat. The flavors are even better the next day.

CHICKEN CRUST JALAPEÑO POPPER PIZZA

This pizza has all the creamy flavor and spice of a jalapeño popper! A cream cheese–based sauce along with crispy bacon make this pizza anything but boring. The crust is packed with protein to keep you full for hours.

Prep time 10 minutes | **Cook time** 40 minutes | **Serves 6**

1 pound ground skinless chicken thigh

½ cup shredded mozzarella

2 tablespoons salted butter

2 ounces cream cheese, softened

½ cup heavy whipping cream

1 cup shredded Monterey jack

⅓ cup sliced pickled jalapeños

4 slices cooked bacon, crumbled

Per Serving
Calories: 375 | Fat: 29g | Protein: 24g | Sodium: 487mg | Fiber: 0g | Carbohydrates: 2g | Net Carbohydrates: 2g | Sugar: 1g

1 Preheat the oven to 400°F. Line a large baking sheet with parchment paper.

2 In a large bowl, mix chicken and mozzarella.

3 Press the chicken mixture into a 10" × 12" rectangle on the prepared baking sheet. Bake for 20 minutes.

4 In a small saucepan over medium heat, melt butter. Whisk in cream cheese and heavy whipping cream until bubbly and smooth, about 1 minute.

5 Sprinkle in Monterey jack and whisk until smooth, about 1 minute. Remove semicooked crust from the oven and top with the cheese sauce, jalapeños, and bacon. Bake for an additional 15 minutes or until cheese is bubbling and chicken crust is fully cooked to at least 165°F internal temperature. Let cool for 5 minutes. Serve warm.

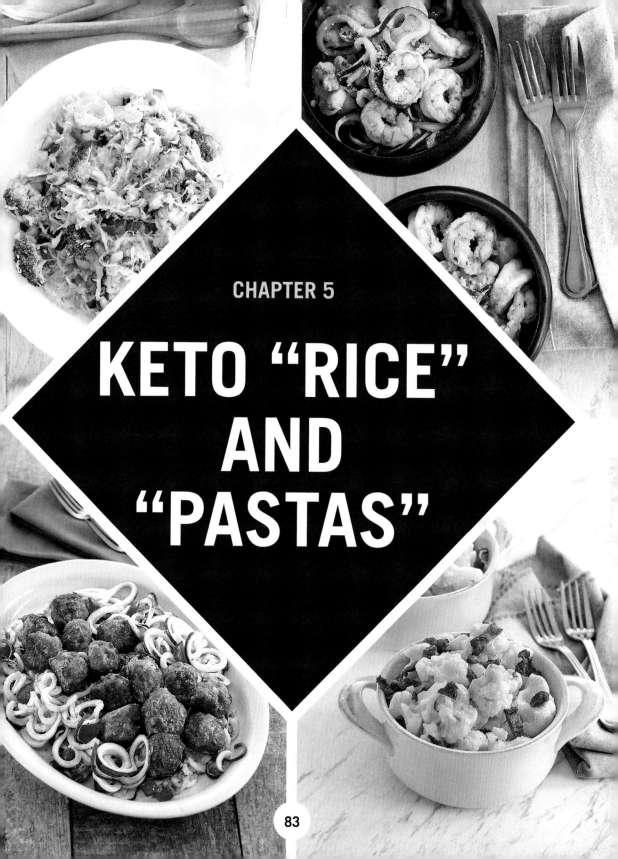

CHAPTER 5

KETO "RICE" AND "PASTAS"

CHEESE-BURGER HELPER

This ultracreamy skillet casserole is a replica of a childhood favorite with more nutrients and fewer carbs than traditional boxed meals. Not only do those meals often use rice or noodles as a base, but they also often have cheese sauces with lots of added fillers and carbs. This meal uses cabbage in place of noodles for texture and a mild taste that absorbs the flavors of the beef. The cabbage and beef come together with a superquick cheese sauce that uses a few ingredients you're likely to already have in the refrigerator. This is sure to be one of your family's weeknight favorites!

Prep time 15 minutes | **Cook time** 35 minutes | **Serves 4**

1 pound 80/20 ground beef
1 teaspoon paprika
½ teaspoon onion powder
¼ teaspoon garlic powder
1 tablespoon tomato paste
¼ cup water
2 cups shredded green cabbage
2 tablespoons salted butter
1 ounce cream cheese, softened
½ cup heavy whipping cream
1½ cups shredded mild Cheddar

Per Serving

Calories: 558 | Fat: 41g | Protein: 31g | Sodium: 458mg | Fiber: 1g | Carbohydrates: 5g | Net Carbohydrates: 4g | Sugar: 2g

1 In a large skillet over medium heat, brown ground beef until no pink remains, about 10 minutes. Drain the excess grease and return the skillet of ground beef to the heat.

2 Add paprika, onion powder, and garlic powder. Stir in tomato paste and water.

3 Place cabbage in the skillet and fold into ground beef. Bring the mixture to a boil and cover. Allow cabbage to cook for 15 minutes or until tender and translucent, stirring occasionally.

4 While cabbage is cooking, prepare the cheese sauce. In a small saucepan over medium heat, melt butter.

5 Whisk in cream cheese and heavy whipping cream until smooth, about 1 minute. The sauce will start to form bubbles; continue whisking and reduce heat to low. Quickly stir in Cheddar.

6 Turn off the heat and continue stirring until all the cheese is melted and the mixture is completely smooth, about 1 minute. (It will be about the thickness of melted Velveeta or queso.)

7 Once cabbage is tender, pour the cheese sauce into the skillet and fold into the ground beef mixture. Serve warm.

MEXICAN-STYLE RICE

This dish is a savory side that perfectly complements any low-carb Mexican dish. Sometimes keto dieters struggle with cauliflower rice as a replacement because the taste isn't similar enough to the real thing. If that's you, give this recipe a try to silence all those doubts. Traditionally, the rice is cooked with tomato sauce, which gives it a red hue. This recipe uses tomato paste, which gives you the same flavor but with fewer carbs. The cilantro and sour cream on top really give it that restaurant-style feel, but if you don't like cilantro feel free to leave it out.

Prep time 10 minutes | **Cook time** 20 minutes | **Serves 4**

3 tablespoons coconut oil

¼ medium yellow onion, peeled and chopped

2 tablespoons tomato paste

1 small serrano pepper, seeded and finely chopped

1 clove garlic, peeled and minced

½ cup chicken broth

1 teaspoon chili powder

1 large head cauliflower, leaves removed, cored, and riced (about 4 cups)

2 tablespoons salted butter

¼ cup fresh cilantro, chopped

¼ cup sour cream

1 In a large skillet over medium heat, melt coconut oil. Add onion and sauté until onion softens and turns translucent, about 3 minutes.

2 Add tomato paste, serrano pepper, and garlic, then stir gently for 1 minute.

3 Pour in the broth then add the chili powder and cauliflower into the pan and allow to cook for 15 minutes until most of the moisture in the pan has evaporated and cauliflower is tender.

4 Remove from heat and fold in butter and cilantro. Serve warm with sour cream.

Per Serving
Calories: 232 | Fat: 18g | Protein: 5g | Sodium: 313mg | Fiber: 5g | Carbohydrates: 14g | Net Carbohydrates: 9g | Sugar: 6g

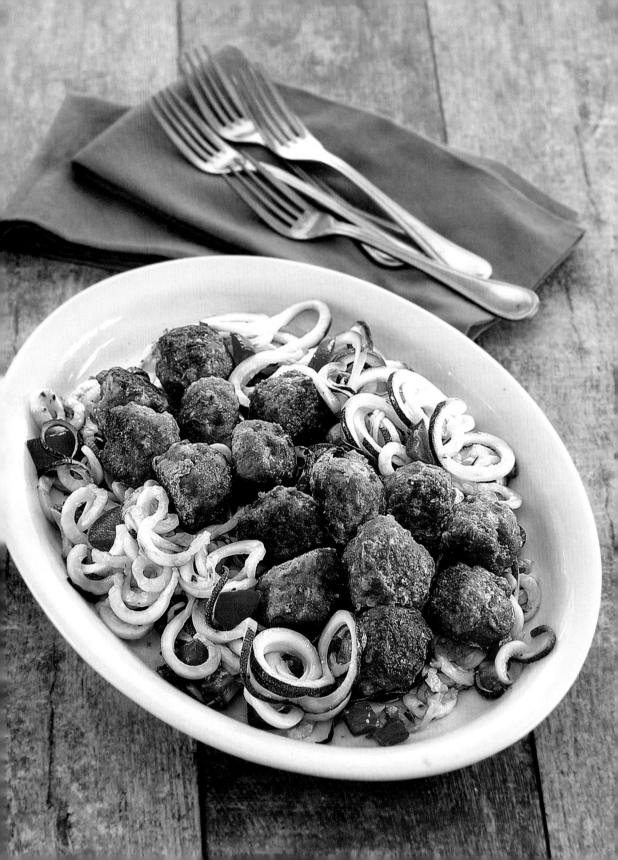

BAKED PESTO CHICKEN MEATBALLS AND ZOODLES

Pesto is great as a sauce, but it also adds a ton of flavor as a mix-in with meat. Its fresh taste makes the perfect complement for chicken to give you a meal that's filling but won't weigh you down. Just look for some keto-friendly pesto at the store. This meal is also perfect as a make-ahead meal. You can double or triple the recipe, bake, then freeze the meatballs to use throughout the month! Just store them in an airtight freezer bag in a single layer for up to 5 months.

Prep time 10 minutes | **Cook time** 30 minutes | **Serves 4**

1 pound ground chicken thigh

¼ cup basil pesto

¼ cup plus 2 tablespoons grated Parmesan, divided

¼ cup shredded mozzarella

¼ teaspoon garlic powder

⅛ teaspoon ground black pepper

2 tablespoons coconut oil

2 tablespoons olive oil

¼ teaspoon dried basil

¼ teaspoon dried oregano

4 medium zucchini, spiralized

½ medium vine tomato, chopped

Per Serving
Calories: 382 | Fat: 28g | Protein: 22g | Sodium: 412mg | Fiber: 2g | Carbohydrates: 10g | Net Carbohydrates: 8g | Sugar: 5g

1 Preheat the oven to 375°F. Line a large baking sheet with parchment paper.

2 In a large bowl, mix chicken, pesto, ¼ cup Parmesan, mozzarella, garlic powder, and pepper. Take about 2 heaping tablespoons of the mixture and form into sixteen balls.

3 In a medium skillet over medium heat, melt coconut oil. Brown the meatballs then transfer to the prepared baking sheet. Bake for 20 minutes or until fully cooked to an internal temperature of at least 165°F.

4 In a large skillet over medium heat, add olive oil, basil, oregano, and zucchini. Cook for 3–5 minutes until zucchini is just beginning to soften. Move to a large bowl and toss with tomatoes. To serve, top zucchini noodles with four meatballs. Sprinkle with the remaining Parmesan.

Make Your Own Ground Chicken

Ground chicken is growing in popularity, but it can still be hard to find in some areas. If you're having trouble finding it, you can use ground chicken breast, which is much more common. You can also place boneless, skinless raw chicken thighs in your food processor or meat grinder and make it yourself!

SPAGHETTI SQUASH AND MEATBALLS

This classic meal gets a low-carb makeover that will get the whole family excited! Pasta is often made of flours that by themselves aren't too flavorful, so they need the help of sauce and herbs. Spaghetti squash has a unique flavor all its own and is only elevated by the seasoning. Though it doesn't taste exactly like spaghetti, you'll get all the savory flavoring found in the traditional meal, and it will be packed with nutrients.

Prep time 10 minutes | **Cook time** 80 minutes | **Serves 4**

1 (4-pound) spaghetti squash

⅛ teaspoon finely ground pink Himalayan salt

⅛ teaspoon ground black pepper

1 cup water

1 pound 80/20 ground beef

¼ cup grated Parmesan

½ teaspoon dried oregano

½ teaspoon dried basil

¼ teaspoon garlic powder

2 tablespoons coconut oil

1 cup low-carb marinara sauce

4 tablespoons salted butter, melted

Per Serving
Calories: 323 | Fat: 19g | Protein: 20g | Sodium: 307mg | Fiber: 3g | Carbohydrates: 14g | Net Carbohydrates: 11g | Sugar: 5g

1 Preheat the oven to 400°F. Line a baking sheet with parchment paper.

2 Poke spaghetti squash with a fork and place on a microwave-safe plate. Microwave for 5 minutes. This will let it soften enough to cut in half. Let it cool completely and cut off the top and bottom. Carefully cut vertically down the center in half. Use a spoon to remove the seeds.

3 Sprinkle squash with salt and pepper, then place into a 9" × 13" baking dish, with skin facing up. Pour water into the dish and bake for 45 minutes, checking intermittently in case of oven hot spots. When done, squash skin will be soft and easily pull away from the inside. Peel and set aside to cool.

4 In a large bowl, mix ground beef, Parmesan, oregano, basil, and garlic powder. Form the mixture into sixteen meatballs. In a medium skillet over medium heat, melt coconut oil. Brown the meatballs for about 7 minutes, then place them on the prepared baking sheet. Bake for 20 minutes or until completely cooked through to at least 160°F.

5 When done, toss meatballs in marinara sauce.

6 Use a fork to pull the strands out of the cooled spaghetti squash. Place them into a bowl, pour in melted butter, and toss.

7 To serve, place 1 cup buttery spaghetti squash on each plate and place four meatballs in the center. Serve warm.

CHICKEN FRIED RICE

This restaurant-inspired meal has it all—flavorful protein and savory vegetables that will have you wishing you doubled the recipe for leftovers. The dish is garlicky with a subtle hint of heat that makes it great for all ages. You can make this dish even faster without compromising flavor by using a rotisserie chicken and steamer bag of cauliflower. This recipe calls for a less fatty cut of chicken, but that doesn't mean it's not a high-fat meal. Fats from the oils add the calories you need, but if you prefer, feel free to swap out breasts for chicken thighs.

Prep time 5 minutes | **Cook time** 30 minutes | **Serves 4**

2 tablespoons coconut oil
¼ medium white onion, peeled and chopped
2 cloves garlic, peeled and finely minced
1 pound chicken breast, cubed
1 cup chicken broth
1 tablespoon sriracha
2 tablespoons soy sauce
1 medium head cauliflower, leaves removed, cored, and riced
2 cups chopped broccoli
2 tablespoons salted butter
1 large egg
1 medium stalk green onion, sliced
1 teaspoon sesame seeds

Per Serving
Calories: 232 | Fat: 16g | Protein: 32g | Sodium: 910mg | Fiber: 5g | Carbohydrates: 13g | Net Carbohydrates: 8g | Sugar: 5g

1 In a large skillet over medium heat, melt coconut oil. Add onion and sauté for 3 minutes or until it begins to soften. Add garlic and sauté for 30 seconds, then add chicken.

2 Allow chicken to sear on each side for 1 minute, then pour in chicken broth and continue cooking until no pink remains in chicken and the internal temperature is at least 165°F, about 15 minutes.

3 Add sriracha, soy sauce, cauliflower, and broccoli to the pan. Reduce the heat to medium-low, cover, and cook for 4–5 minutes or until the broccoli is crisp yet tender.

4 Place butter in the pan and allow to melt and stir in with chicken and vegetables, about 1 minute.

5 Push the rice to the edges of the pan and leave a hole in the center of the pan. Crack open egg into the center and allow it to firm up, about 1 minute, then flip it and chop it up with a spatula. Fold egg into the rest of the mixture.

6 Garnish with green onion and sesame seeds. Serve warm.

BAKED BACON CAULIFLOWER MAC AND CHEESE

If you have picky eaters in your home, this cheesy dish is one of the best ways to introduce keto meal options. This is a great recipe for those who are new to cooking cauliflower because it's made with steamer bags, so it cooks quickly and with no effort.

Prep time 5 minutes | **Cook time** 35 minutes | **Serves 6**

2 (12-ounce) steamer bags cauliflower florets

4 tablespoons salted butter

¼ medium yellow onion, peeled and diced

2 ounces cream cheese, softened

½ cup heavy whipping cream

1½ cups shredded sharp Cheddar

6 slices cooked bacon, crumbled

Per Serving
Calories: 365 | Fat: 29g | Protein: 14g | Sodium: 505mg | Fiber: 3g | Carbohydrates: 7g | Net Carbohydrates: 4g | Sugar: 4g

1 Preheat the oven to 400°F.

2 Cook cauliflower according to package instructions. Open bags and allow to cool completely. Wring out excess moisture in a kitchen towel or cheesecloth and place cauliflower into a large bowl.

3 In a large skillet over medium heat, melt butter. Add onion and sauté for 3 minutes until it softens. In a small bowl, whisk cream cheese and heavy whipping cream together. Pour the mixture into the skillet.

4 Sprinkle Cheddar into the skillet and quickly whisk until a smooth cheese sauce forms. Add cauliflower and fold into the cheese sauce until completely covered, about 1 minute.

5 Transfer the mixture into an 8" × 8" baking dish and bake for 10 minutes. Remove from oven to sprinkle bacon over the top and then return to the oven for an additional 10 minutes or until bubbling and the top begins to turn golden brown. Allow 10 minutes to cool. Serve warm.

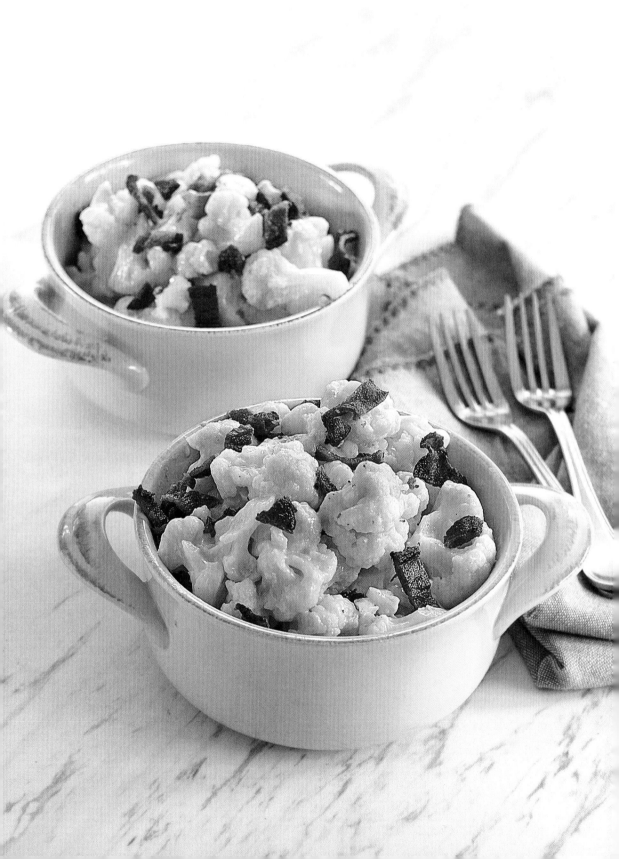

PASTA PRIMAVERA

There are lots of low-carb vegetable options that you can enjoy in moderation, such as bell peppers and cruciferous vegetables. This dish highlights those bright tastes alongside a high-fat creamy sauce and keto-friendly noodles.

Prep time 5 minutes | **Cook time** 65 minutes | **Serves 4**

1 (4-pound) spaghetti squash
2 cups water
2 tablespoons olive oil
1 medium zucchini, chopped
1 cup chopped broccoli
¼ medium red bell pepper, seeded and chopped
⅛ teaspoon ground black pepper
⅛ teaspoon finely ground pink Himalayan salt
4 tablespoons salted butter
¼ cup heavy whipping cream
½ cup grated Parmesan

Per Serving
Calories: 335 | Fat: 26g | Protein: 7g | Sodium: 417mg | Fiber: 4g | Carbohydrates: 18g | Net Carbohydrates: 14g | Sugar: 7g

1 Preheat the oven to 400°F.

2 Use a fork to poke holes in spaghetti squash and place it on a microwave-safe plate. Microwave for 5 minutes, then let cool for 5 minutes.

3 Carefully cut the ends off squash and cut squash vertically into two halves. Use a spoon to remove the seeds.

4 Pour water into a 9" × 13" baking dish and place squash halves skin-side up into the pan. Bake for 50 minutes or until tender. Use a fork to remove the strands and place them into a large bowl.

5 In a large skillet over medium heat, warm olive oil. Add zucchini, broccoli, bell pepper, black pepper, and salt.

6 Sauté the vegetables for 7 minutes until all are fork-tender. Place them into the bowl with the spaghetti squash strands.

7 In a large saucepan over medium heat, melt butter. Pour in heavy whipping cream and whisk in Parmesan. Bring to a boil and then reduce, cooking for 2 minutes until the mixture begins to thicken.

8 Add spaghetti squash strands and cooked vegetables to the sauce and toss to coat. Serve warm.

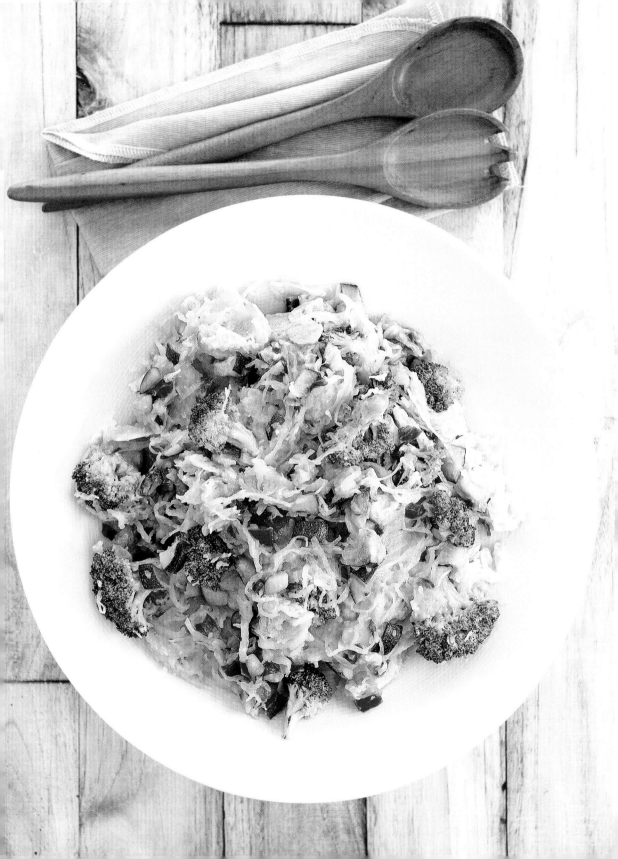

CILANTRO LIME CAULIFLOWER RICE

This side dish comes together quickly and pairs perfectly with any protein! Whether you're making a burrito bowl or you need some extra vegetables alongside your protein, this rice is buttery with a hint of sour from the lime that brightens up any meal. To save even more time, you can use a steamer bag of cauliflower rice!

Prep time 5 minutes | **Cook time** 20 minutes | **Serves 4**

1 large head cauliflower
2 tablespoons coconut oil
1 clove garlic, peeled and finely minced
1 small lime, juiced and zested
⅓ cup vegetable broth
2 tablespoons salted butter, melted
½ cup chopped fresh cilantro
½ teaspoon finely ground pink Himalayan salt
⅛ teaspoon ground black pepper

Per Serving
Calories: 149 | Fat: 12g | Protein: 3g | Sodium: 330mg | Fiber: 3g | Carbohydrates: 8g | Net Carbohydrates: 5g | Sugar: 3g

1 Remove the leaves and core from cauliflower. Cut cauliflower into florets and place into a food processor. Pulse about ten times or until cauliflower is rice-like.

2 In a large skillet over medium heat, melt coconut oil. Add garlic and stir until fragrant, about 30 seconds. Pour in lime juice and zest and vegetable broth.

3 Add cauliflower to the pan and stir until evenly coated with broth. Continue cooking for 15 minutes or until it becomes soft and most of the moisture has evaporated, stirring occasionally.

4 Pour butter over cauliflower and gently fold in cilantro, salt, and pepper. Serve warm.

Make It a Bowl

Use this rice as a base for a burrito bowl. Top with grilled chicken, sautéed vegetables, Monterey jack, guacamole, and sour cream for a quick, meal-prep-friendly lunch! It will also taste good mixed with chili or added to soup for an extra-filling meal.

ROASTED SPAGHETTI SQUASH CARBONARA

Carbonara is perfect for a keto diet because it's naturally high in fat. This dish takes advantage of the cheesy flavor and keeps it close to the classic by swapping only the noodles for a lower-carb option. Although spaghetti squash takes longer to cook than regular pasta, it contains vitamin C, vitamin A, and fiber!

Prep time 5 minutes | **Cook time** 70 minutes | **Serves 4**

1 (4-pound) spaghetti squash

2 cups water

6 slices bacon

4 tablespoons salted butter

⅛ teaspoon ground black pepper

⅛ teaspoon pink Himalayan salt

2 large egg yolks

1 large egg

1 cup grated Parmesan

1 tablespoon chopped fresh parsley

Per Serving
Calories: 384 | Fat: 26g | Protein: 17g | Sodium: 938mg | Fiber: 3g | Carbohydrates: 17g | Net Carbohydrates: 14g | Sugar: 5g

1 Preheat the oven to 400°F.

2 Use a fork to poke holes in spaghetti squash, then place it on a microwave-safe plate. Microwave for 5 minutes or until tender enough to cut. Allow it to cool for 5 minutes.

3 Slice the ends off squash, then cut it vertically down the center. Use a spoon to remove the seeds.

4 Place the two halves, skin-side up, in a 9" × 13" baking dish. Pour water into the bottom of the dish. Bake for 40–50 minutes or until tender. Allow it to cool, then use a fork to separate the strands.

5 In a large skillet over medium heat, fry bacon until crispy, about 10 minutes. Place it aside on paper towels to cool, then crumble. Drain the grease from the pan and return the pan to medium heat. Add butter. Place the squash strands into the pan and sprinkle with pepper and salt.

6 In a small bowl, whisk egg yolks, egg, and Parmesan together. Pour the mixture over squash and toss for 3 minutes continuously until fully coated. A light but creamy sauce will form. Sprinkle in crumbled bacon. Remove from the heat and allow 3 minutes to cool. Garnish with parsley. Serve warm.

SHRIMP SCAMPI WITH ZOODLES

Shrimp is a great seafood option for the keto diet because it has virtually no carbs, but it is a good source of omega-3 fatty acids, healthy fats that help keep your heart healthy. Be sure to use fresh shrimp over the frozen, precooked variety to experience even greater flavor.

Prep time 10 minutes | **Cook time** 15 minutes | **Serves 4**

3 tablespoons salted butter

2 tablespoons olive oil

2 cloves garlic, peeled and minced

¼ teaspoon finely ground pink Himalayan salt

⅛ teaspoon ground black pepper

⅛ teaspoon crushed red pepper flakes

1 pound medium shrimp, shelled and deveined

¼ cup lemon juice

¼ cup chicken broth

4 medium zucchini, spiralized

¼ cup grated Parmesan

Per Serving

Calories: 269 | Fat: 17g | Protein: 18g | Sodium: 846mg | Fiber: 2g | Carbohydrates: 10g | Net Carbohydrates: 9g | Sugar: 5g

1 In a large skillet over medium heat, melt butter. Drizzle olive oil in the pan. Sauté garlic until fragrant, about 30 seconds.

2 Sprinkle salt, black pepper, and red pepper flakes on shrimp, then place into the pan and sauté for 3 minutes until shrimp is pink and beginning to curl. Remove shrimp from the pan and set aside to prevent overcooking.

3 Pour lemon juice and broth into the pan, whisk together, and let the liquid reduce by a third, about 4 minutes.

4 Add zucchini to the pan and toss to coat. Let cook for 3–4 minutes until it begins to soften a little. (Overcooking will result in soggy noodles.)

5 Add shrimp back to the pan and toss. Sprinkle with Parmesan. Serve warm.

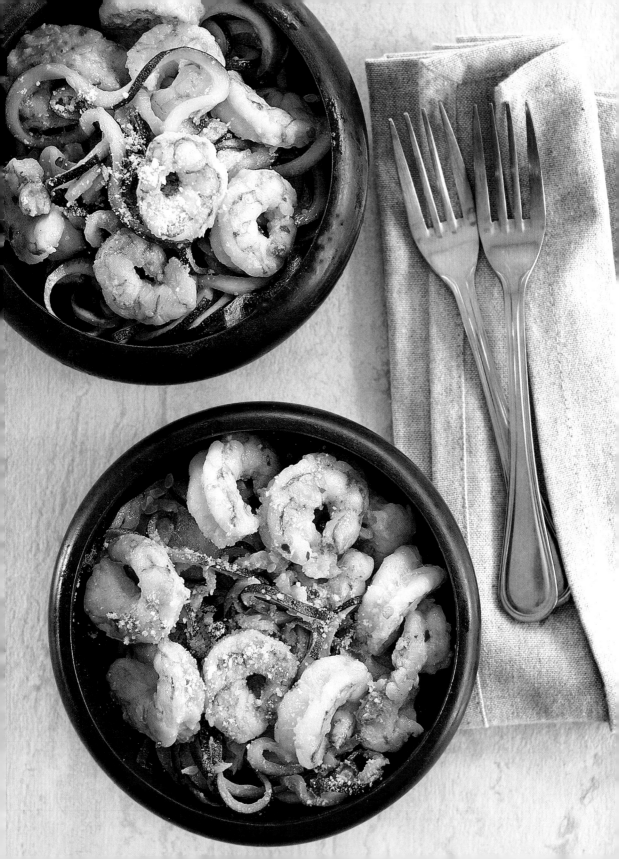

CUCUMBER RANCH SALAD

Traditional pasta salads are full of noodles on top of high-fat sauces—which makes for a high-calorie side dish! This recipe trades the noodles for crisp cucumbers, which brings the calories and carbs way down, but it still keeps the delicious and creamy sauce. Feel free to get creative and add your favorite vegetables.

Prep time 10 minutes | **Cook time** N/A | **Serves 8**

¼ cup mayonnaise

¼ cup sour cream

2 tablespoons dry ranch seasoning

6 medium cucumbers, spiralized

½ cup sliced grape tomatoes

4 slices cooked bacon, chopped

2 tablespoons diced peeled red onion

Per Serving
Calories: 118 | Fat: 8g | Protein: 3g | Sodium: 349mg | Fiber: 1g | Carbohydrates: 8g | Net Carbohydrates: 7g | Sugar: 3g

In a large bowl, whisk mayonnaise, sour cream, and ranch seasoning. Gently fold the remaining ingredients into the sauce until evenly coated. Chill for at least 30 minutes before serving.

MUSHROOM "WILD RICE"

This dish is a low-carb spin on a midwestern favorite, where wild rice grows abundantly. The earthy flavor from the mushrooms paired with the herbs create a warm and comforting dish to enjoy as a side, or combine it with some chicken for a hearty meal. The texture is softer than traditional rice, but you'll still get that "riced" mushroom taste as well as a little crunchy texture from the celery.

Prep time 10 minutes | **Cook time** 10 minutes | **Serves 4**

1 cup cremini mushrooms

1 medium stalk celery, chopped

⅓ medium carrot, peeled and diced

2 tablespoons salted butter

2 tablespoons olive oil

1 clove garlic, peeled and finely minced

½ teaspoon dried thyme

¼ teaspoon finely ground pink Himalayan salt

½ cup hemp hearts

⅓ cup chicken broth

2 tablespoons chopped fresh parsley

Per Serving
Calories: 234 | Fat: 21g | Protein: 8g | Sodium: 233mg | Fiber: 1g | Carbohydrates: 4g | Net Carbohydrates: 3g | Sugar: 1g

1 In a food processor, pulse mushrooms, celery, and carrot until mushrooms are small and rice-like, about 30 seconds.

2 In a medium skillet over medium heat, warm butter and olive oil, about 30 seconds. Add the vegetable mixture to the pan and sprinkle with garlic, thyme, and salt. Sauté until the vegetables begin to soften, 2–3 minutes.

3 Pour hemp hearts and broth in the pan. Simmer for 2–3 minutes until seeds absorb moisture. Fluff with a fork, then garnish with parsley. Serve warm.

Where Do I Find Hemp Hearts?

You can usually find hemp hearts in the baking section of your local grocery store near the flaxseed, but you may need to check in the health section. They can be used in savory dishes like this one but can also be a great addition to low-carb granola or smoothies. Hemp hearts are a good source of fiber and iron as well as protein. They have fewer carbs and more protein than flax or chia seeds, which make them a great alternative.

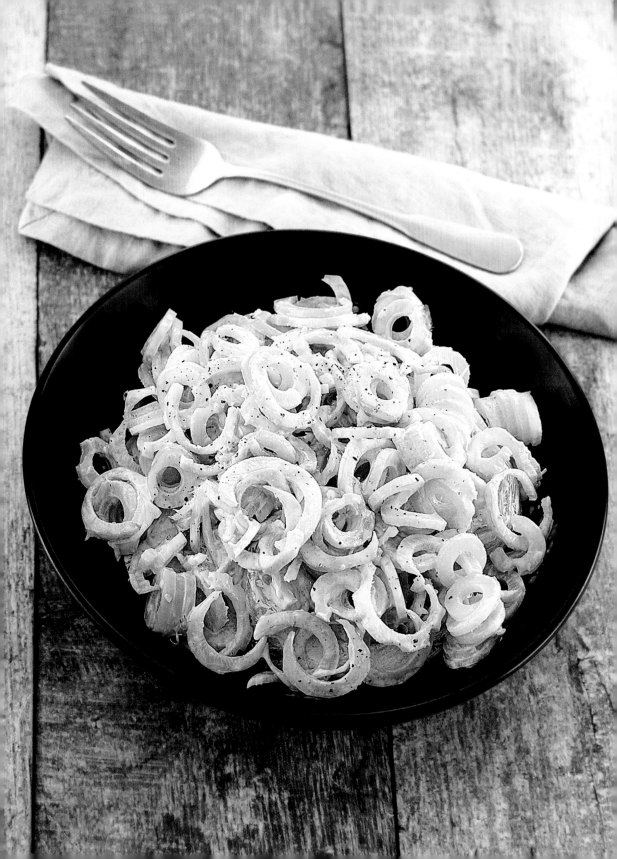

SPIRALIZED BROCCOLI ALFREDO

Spiralizing isn't just for squash! Don't let those broccoli stems go to waste—slice them and use them as noodles. The classic dish just adds a few florets of broccoli alongside lots of pasta, but this low-carb swap makes the vegetables the star. Feel free to add your favorite protein for an even more filling meal.

Prep time 10 minutes | **Cook time** 15 minutes | **Serves 2**

4 large broccoli stems
4 tablespoons salted butter
¼ medium yellow onion, peeled and diced
2 ounces cream cheese, softened
½ cup heavy whipping cream
¼ cup chicken broth
⅛ teaspoon ground black pepper
⅛ teaspoon finely ground pink Himalayan salt
½ cup shredded Parmesan

Per Serving
Calories: 340 | Fat: 29g | Protein: 9g | Sodium: 465mg | Fiber: 0g | Carbohydrates: 10g | Net Carbohydrates: 10g | Sugar: 2g

1 Spiralize broccoli stems. In a medium pot over medium heat, bring 2 cups water to a boil. Place spiralized stems in a steamer basket and carefully place it into the boiling water. Place the lid on the pot and let steam for 5 minutes. Remove and set aside to cool.

2 In a medium skillet over medium heat, melt butter. Add onion and sauté until softened, about 3 minutes. Whisk in cream cheese, heavy whipping cream, and broth. Bring to a boil, then reduce the heat to low to simmer until the mixture begins to reduce and thicken, about 4 minutes.

3 Sprinkle in pepper, salt, and Parmesan. Whisk until smooth, about 30 seconds. Add spiralized stems into the pan and toss to coat. Serve warm.

Use All Parts of Broccoli

If you don't have time to spiralize, you can slice up the stems or even enjoy florets in the meal! Broccoli stems have almost the same nutritional value as the tops: They're an excellent source of both vitamin C and vitamin A.

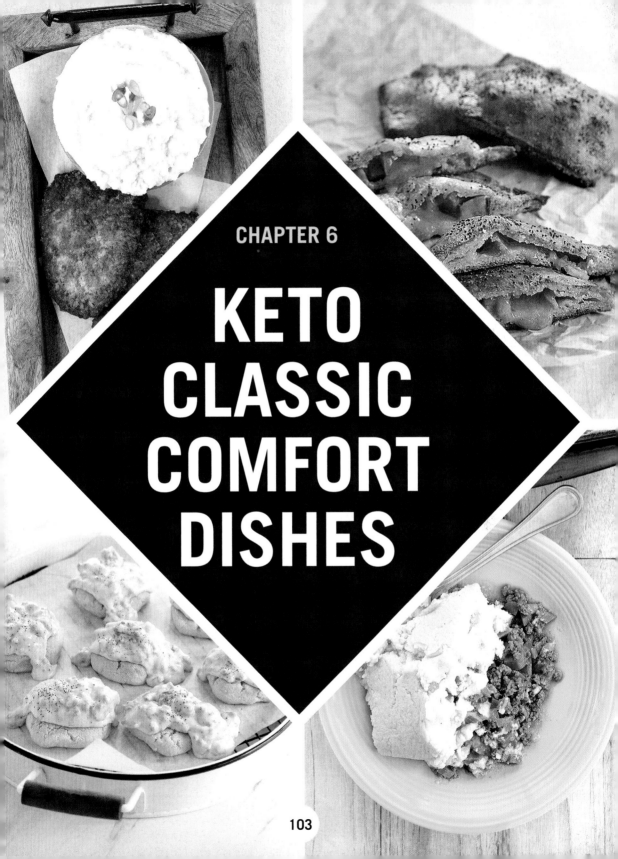

CHAPTER 6

KETO CLASSIC COMFORT DISHES

BISCUITS AND GRAVY

Nothing says a comforting breakfast quite like Biscuits and Gravy. This southern classic with a low-carb spin will remind you of days gone by, especially on those cold and rainy nothing-to-do days. If you love fluffy, buttery biscuits and creamy gravy, you're going to be making double batches of this!

Prep time 10 minutes | **Cook time** 40 minutes | **Serves 6**

2 cups finely ground blanched almond flour

2 teaspoons baking powder

4 tablespoons unsalted butter, softened

½ teaspoon apple cider vinegar

¼ teaspoon finely ground pink Himalayan salt

2 large eggs

1 pound ground pork breakfast sausage

2 tablespoons salted butter

2 ounces cream cheese, softened

½ cup heavy whipping cream

½ cup chicken broth

⅛ teaspoon xanthan gum

¼ teaspoon ground black pepper

Per Serving
Calories: 671 | Fat: 59g | Protein: 23g | Sodium: 892mg | Fiber: 4g | Carbohydrates: 9g | Net Carbohydrates: 5g | Sugar: 3g

1 Preheat the oven to 350°F. Line a baking sheet with parchment paper.

2 In a large bowl, mix almond flour and baking powder. Then, mix in butter, vinegar, salt, and eggs. Allow the mixture to sit for 5 minutes before scooping into ten mounds on the prepared baking sheet.

3 Bake for 10–12 minutes until edges become golden and crispy. Allow to cool for 10 minutes to firm up.

4 In a medium skillet over medium-low heat, cook sausage for 5 minutes. (Cooking low first will render the fat, which will create the sauce.) Increase to medium heat and finish cooking sausage until no pink remains, about 10 minutes.

5 Add butter to the pan and whisk in cream cheese. Pour in heavy whipping cream and broth and whisk until smooth, then add xanthan gum and pepper. Whisk quickly to allow xanthan gum to thicken up the mixture. Continue cooking for 10 minutes until the mixture is thicker and gravy-like. Serve warm over biscuits.

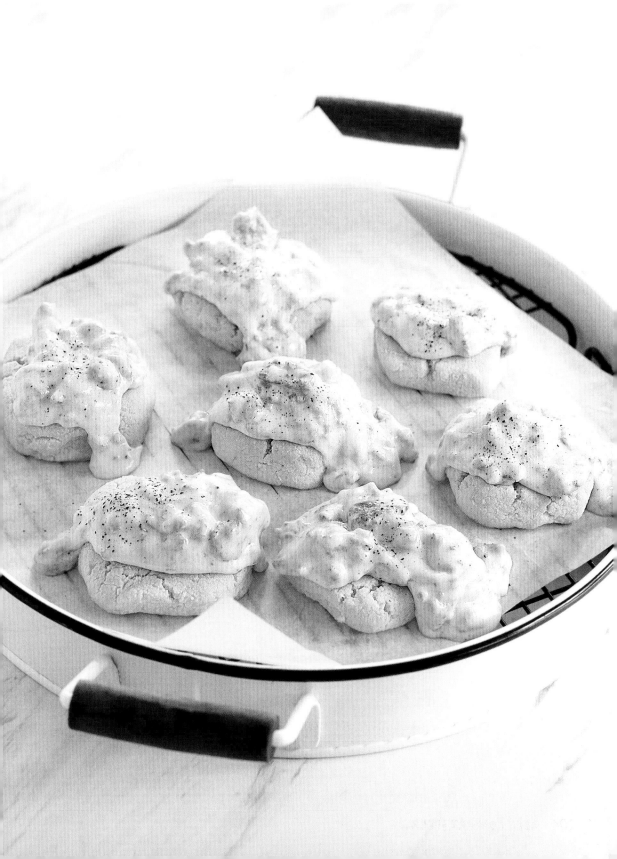

MEATLOAF

There's nothing quite like homemade Meatloaf. Despite the fact that most recipes use bread crumbs as a binder, you truly don't need them. This Meatloaf will stay together with the help of mayonnaise, which also keeps it moist. You also have to avoid the sugary glaze used in the classic version—but don't worry, erythritol can caramelize too!

Prep time 10 minutes | **Cook time** 50 minutes | **Serves 4**

1 pound 80/20 ground beef

1 large egg

¼ cup mayonnaise

½ medium yellow onion, peeled and chopped

2 ounces plain pork rinds, finely ground

½ cup shredded mild Cheddar

¼ teaspoon finely ground pink Himalayan salt

⅛ teaspoon ground black pepper

¼ teaspoon garlic powder

⅛ teaspoon dried oregano

⅛ teaspoon dried basil

2 tablespoons tomato paste

1 tablespoon salted butter

1 teaspoon granular erythritol

¼ cup water

Per Serving

Calories: 575 | Fat: 42g | Protein: 33g | Sodium: 687mg | Fiber: 1g | Carbohydrates: 5g | Sugar Alcohol: 1g | Net Carbohydrates: 4g | Sugar: 2g

1 Preheat the oven to 400°F.

2 In a large bowl, mix all ingredients except tomato paste, butter, erythritol, and water. Place the mixture into a 9" × 5" loaf pan and form into a loaf.

3 In a small saucepan over medium heat, whisk tomato paste, butter, erythritol, and water. Bring to a boil at medium, then reduce the heat to simmer over low and allow it to simmer for 3–5 minutes until it begins to thicken.

4 Pour the tomato sauce over the meatloaf, then cover the pan with foil and bake for 45 minutes. Remove the foil halfway through the cook time. Meatloaf will be fully cooked when it reaches at least 160°F. Let cool for at least 5 minutes before slicing. Serve warm.

Add a Barbecue-Flavored Twist!

If you're a fan of barbecue flavors, swap out the tomato paste topping for barbecue sauce! Check the health section of your local grocery store to find low-carb sauce options. Ken Davis Sassy 2 Carb sauce is sweetened with sucralose and is thick like traditional sauce.

STROGANOFF

Stroganoff is one of the top American comfort foods, but did you know that this stew-like dish originated in Russia? Although its main ingredients—beef and sour cream—are totally keto-friendly, it is often served over pasta. Once you swap that out for nutritious and filling cabbage, you have an irresistible comfort stew that your family won't be able to get enough of!

Prep time 10 minutes | **Cook time** 50 minutes | **Serves 4**

2 tablespoons coconut oil

⅛ teaspoon ground black pepper

¼ teaspoon finely ground pink Himalayan salt

1 pound sirloin steak, sliced in 2" strips

4 tablespoons salted butter, cubed

4 ounces cremini mushrooms, sliced

¼ medium yellow onion, peeled and diced

1 clove garlic, peeled and minced

¾ cup beef broth

2 ounces cream cheese, softened

1 cup sour cream

½ teaspoon xanthan gum

2 teaspoons olive oil

4 cups shredded green cabbage

Per Serving
Calories: 598 | Fat: 46g | Protein: 27g | Sodium: 510mg | Fiber: 2g | Carbohydrates: 9g | Net Carbohydrates: 7g | Sugar: 3g

1 In a large skillet over medium heat, melt coconut oil. Sprinkle pepper and salt over the steak, then sear steak until no pink remains, about 5 minutes per side.

2 Add butter to the pan and stir in until melted. Add mushrooms, onion, and garlic. Cook for 3–5 minutes or until mushrooms soften, stirring occasionally.

3 Pour broth into the pan and let simmer for 20 minutes, stirring occasionally, letting the mixture reduce by half.

4 In a small bowl, whisk cream cheese and sour cream together. Stir the mixture into the pan and sprinkle in xanthan gum and stir, allowing the mixture to thicken for 4–5 minutes.

5 In a medium skillet over medium heat, warm olive oil. Sauté cabbage until softened and translucent, about 12 minutes.

6 To serve, top cabbage with meat sauce. Serve warm.

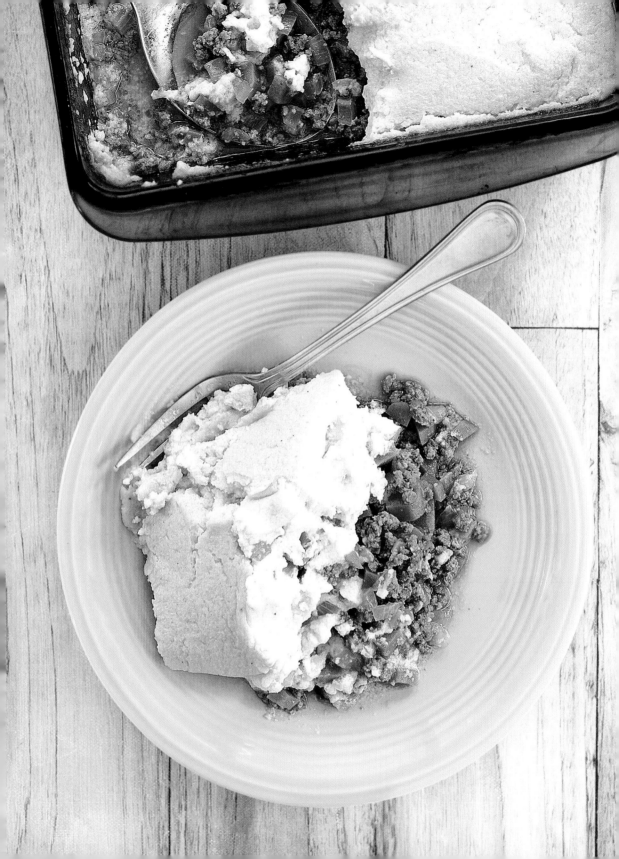

SHEPHERD'S PIE

Each spoonful of this hearty meal will give you a perfectly well-rounded, savory bite. The creamy, cheesy mashed cauliflower is a flavorful spin on the classic mashed potatoes that you'll wish you had tried sooner.

Prep time 30 minutes | **Cook time** 60 minutes | **Serves 4**

1 pound 80/20 ground beef

2 tablespoons salted butter

½ medium white onion, peeled and diced

2 large carrots, peeled and diced

1 medium stalk celery, chopped

½ cup beef broth

2 (12-ounce) steamer bags cauliflower

2 ounces cream cheese

1 cup shredded sharp Cheddar

¼ cup sour cream

¼ teaspoon finely ground pink Himalayan salt

¼ teaspoon garlic powder

⅛ teaspoon ground black pepper

Per Serving

Calories: 319 | Fat: 20g | Protein: 19g | Sodium: 345mg | Fiber: 4g | Carbohydrates: 10g | Net Carbohydrates: 6g | Sugar: 5g

1 Preheat the oven to 375°F.

2 In a large pot over medium heat, brown ground beef until no pink remains, about 10 minutes. Drain the excess fat and return beef over medium heat.

3 Place butter into the pot, then add onion. Add carrots and celery and sauté for 5 minutes or until carrots begin to soften.

4 Pour in beef broth, then simmer for 15 minutes or until vegetables are tender and liquid reduces by half.

5 Microwave cauliflower according to the package instructions, about 5 minutes, then place into a food processor. Add cream cheese, Cheddar, sour cream, salt, garlic powder, and pepper. Pulse until smooth and creamy, about ten pulses, scraping down the sides as needed.

6 Pour the beef mixture into an 8" × 8" casserole dish. Carefully spoon the mashed cauliflower on top and bake for 20 minutes or until bubbly. Let cool for 10 minutes. Serve warm.

CRISPY AVOCADO FRY NACHOS

Gooey, cheesy nachos loaded with flavorful toppings are the ultimate crowd-pleasing dish. This recipe is perfect for game day, movie night, or whenever the craving hits for a Mexican-style treat. Instead of pork rinds, which are typical in keto diet nacho recipes, this recipe uses avocado fries. Avocados are of course the main ingredient in guacamole, making their inclusion even more perfect, but they're also an incredible source of healthy fats. This recipe uses slightly underripe avocados, so your fries won't be mushy—they'll be creamy inside with a big crunch on the outside.

Prep time 10 minutes | **Cook time** 30 minutes | **Serves 4**

1 large egg

6 ounces 100% Parmesan cheese crisps, crushed

2 medium slightly underripe avocados, peeled, pitted, and sliced into ¼" slices (about 6 slices per avocado half)

1 pound 80/20 ground beef

¼ cup water

½ tablespoon chili powder

½ teaspoon ground cumin

2 teaspoons paprika

¼ teaspoon garlic powder

¼ teaspoon dried oregano

¼ teaspoon ground black pepper

⅛ teaspoon finely ground pink Himalayan salt

1 cup shredded mild Cheddar

2 cups shredded romaine lettuce

4 tablespoons sour cream

1 medium stalk green onion, sliced

1 Preheat the oven to 400°F. Line a large baking sheet with parchment paper.

2 Whisk egg in a medium bowl. Place cheese crisps in a large bowl.

3 Dip each slice of avocado in egg, press gently into cheese crisps to mostly coat, then place onto the prepared baking sheet. Bake for 14 minutes, flipping halfway through. Set aside to cool completely.

4 In a medium skillet over medium heat, brown ground beef until no pink remains, about 10 minutes. Drain the excess grease, then return the skillet to the heat. Pour in water, then sprinkle in chili powder, cumin, paprika, garlic powder, oregano, pepper, and salt. Stir to combine all seasonings with ground beef. Reduce heat to a simmer over low and continue cooking for 4–5 minutes until most of the water is evaporated.

5 To prepare the nachos, place six avocado fries in a circle, then top with ¼ taco beef, ¼ cup Cheddar, ½ cup romaine lettuce, 1 tablespoon sour cream, and garnish with green onion. Serve warm.

Per Serving

Calories: 574 | Fat: 39g | Protein: 39g | Sodium: 871mg | Fiber: 6g | Carbohydrates: 10g | Net Carbohydrates: 4g | Sugar: 1g

CHICKEN TORTILLA ENCHILADAS

Instead of using a traditional tortilla, this recipe uses chicken, eliminating a huge bulk of carbs from the traditional recipe. The protein will help keep you full and strong. With nutrition like this, you'll feel comfortable coming back for seconds!

Prep time 15 minutes | **Cook time** 15 minutes | **Serves 4**

2 cups shredded cooked chicken thigh

1½ cups low-carb green enchilada sauce, divided

1½ cups shredded Monterey jack, divided

16 (½-ounce, thin-sliced) slices deli chicken

1 avocado, peeled, pitted, and sliced

½ cup sour cream

¼ cup chopped fresh cilantro

Per Serving
Calories: 488 | Fat: 30g | Protein: 39g | Sodium: 1,359mg | Fiber: 2g | Carbohydrates: 11g | Net Carbohydrates: 9g | Sugar: 3g

1 Preheat the oven to 400°F.

2 In a large bowl, mix shredded chicken, ½ cup enchilada sauce, and 1 cup Monterey jack.

3 On a work surface, place two slices deli chicken on top of each other. Place about 4 tablespoons of the chicken mixture in the center. Roll and place into an 8" × 8" baking dish. Repeat with the remaining ingredients to make eight rolls total.

4 Pour the remaining sauce over the rolls and sprinkle with the remaining Monterey jack. Bake for 15 minutes or until cheese is melted.

5 Top each serving with ¼ avocado and 2 tablespoons sour cream. Garnish with cilantro. Serve warm.

COUNTRY FRIED STEAK

Steak is a great source of protein and is naturally higher in fat than leaner proteins such as chicken. This recipe takes the classic and gives it a low-carb twist by using a mixture of pork rinds and protein powder. You can complete this meal by adding Mashed Cauliflower and Gravy (see recipe in Chapter 7) and some keto Dinner Rolls (see recipe in Chapter 8) for a delicious meal that doesn't feel low in carbs!

Prep time 15 minutes | **Cook time** 15 minutes | **Serves 4**

¼ cup coconut oil

1 large egg

¼ cup crushed plain pork rinds

¼ cup unflavored protein powder

4 (⅓-pound) cube steaks, tenderized

⅛ teaspoon finely ground sea salt

⅛ teaspoon ground black pepper

1 In a large skillet over medium-high heat, melt coconut oil. Whisk egg in a medium bowl.

2 In a large bowl, mix pork rinds and protein powder. Sprinkle steak with salt and pepper.

3 Dip each steak into egg and then dredge in the pork-rind mixture. Carefully drop each steak into the sizzling oil and fry for 5–7 minutes per side until dark and golden. Place steak on paper towels to absorb the excess oil and cool for 5 minutes. Serve warm.

Per Serving
Calories: 338 | Fat: 13g | Protein: 55g | Sodium: 335mg | Fiber: 0g | Carbohydrates: 0g | Net Carbohydrates: 0g | Sugar: 0g

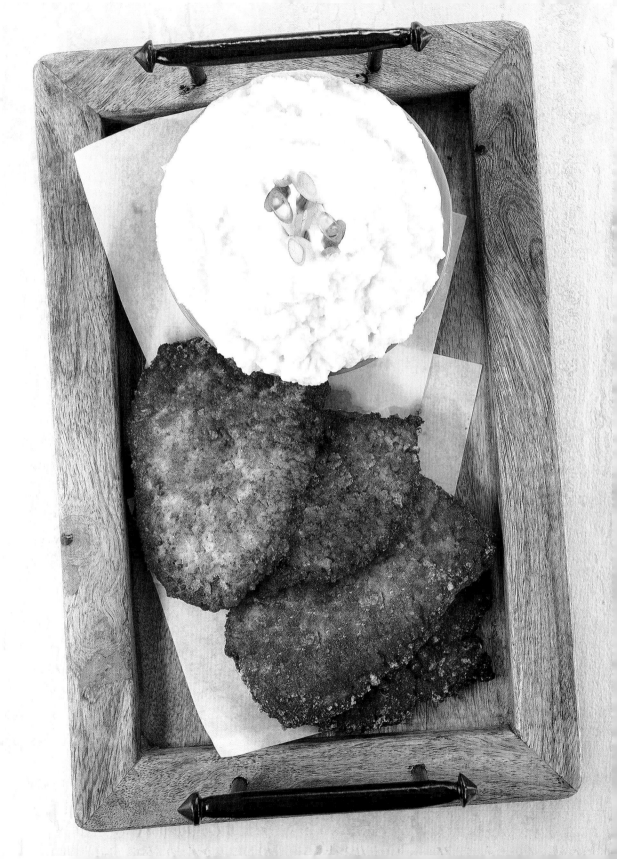

PICKLE-BRINED CRISPY CHICKEN

Want to know the secret to perfectly crispy chicken that keeps all of its juicy favor? Pickle juice! Marinating your chicken in this salty juice adds a ton of flavor. Sometimes frying the outside leaves the inside a bit dry and bland, but the sour cream adds a layer of protection to make sure your fried chicken is crispy on the outside and moist in the center. This recipe bakes the chicken first, then gives it a quick fry for an extracrispy coating that won't fall off.

Prep time 45 minutes | **Cook time** 30 minutes | **Serves 4**

1 pound boneless, skinless chicken tenders

1 cup dill pickle juice

½ cup sour cream

2 ounces plain pork rinds, finely ground

½ cup unflavored, no-sugar-added protein powder

2 large eggs

½ teaspoon ground black pepper

½ teaspoon finely ground finely ground pink Himalayan salt

¼ teaspoon garlic powder

¼ teaspoon onion powder

¼ teaspoon cayenne powder

2 tablespoons coconut oil

Per Serving
Calories: 317 | Fat: 12g | Protein: 49g | Sodium: 766mg | Fiber: 0g | Carbohydrates: 1g | Net Carbohydrates: 1g | Sugar: 0g

1 Place chicken in a large bowl. In a medium bowl, whisk pickle juice and sour cream together. Pour the mixture over chicken and cover bowl with plastic wrap. Marinate for 30 minutes in the refrigerator.

2 Preheat the oven to 400°F. Line a large baking sheet with parchment paper.

3 Mix pork rinds and protein powder in a separate large bowl. Whisk eggs in a clean medium bowl.

4 Sprinkle chicken with pepper, salt, garlic powder, onion powder, and cayenne. Dip chicken in egg, then dredge in the pork-rind mixture. Place onto the prepared baking sheet. Bake for 25 minutes.

5 In a large skillet over medium heat, melt coconut oil. Place each piece of chicken into the hot oil for 45 seconds–1 minute on each side until golden brown. Let cool for 5 minutes before serving.

High-Protein Meals

To balance out the higher protein in this meal, plan ahead during the day to make sure this fits your macros. To add more fat, you can add your favorite high-fat dipping sauce (such as ranch), which will give this recipe an immediate fat boost.

NAKED OVEN-FRIED CHICKEN WINGS

These wings are just as crispy and delicious as the ones you'd order from a restaurant. But with no breading on the outside or oil to fry them in, they're also much better for you. The flavoring possibilities are endless too: Toss them in buffalo sauce, sprinkle on some lemon pepper seasoning, or enjoy them dipped in ranch. No matter which direction you take, these wings will always hit the spot!

Prep time 10 minutes | **Cook time** 85 minutes | **Serves 4**

2 pounds chicken wings, cut into drumettes and flats

1 tablespoon baking powder

¼ teaspoon ground black pepper

½ teaspoon finely ground pink Himalayan salt

4 tablespoons salted butter

Per Serving
Calories: 544 | Fat: 41g | Protein: 40g | Sodium: 842mg | Fiber: 1g | Carbohydrates: 3g | Net Carbohydrates: 2g | Sugar: 0g

1 Preheat the oven to 275°F.

2 Toss wings in a large bowl with baking powder.

3 Place wings on two large baking sheets with a rack, with at least 1" of space between. Sprinkle half of pepper and salt over the wings, then flip and sprinkle the remaining amounts on the other sides.

4 Bake for 30 minutes. Then increase the heat to 400°F and bake for 45–50 minutes or until completely cooked through to an internal temperature of at least 165°F.

5 Melt butter in a large microwave-safe bowl for 30 seconds and toss wings until coated. Serve warm.

The Secret to Crispy Oven Wings

This recipe uses baking powder to get the wings extracrunchy. Since these wings aren't breaded, there's no flour to react with. Instead, the baking powder reacts with the chicken wing skin and changes its pH. The low-temperature cooking renders the fat slowly under the skin before the higher temperature and change in pH makes supercrispy wings!

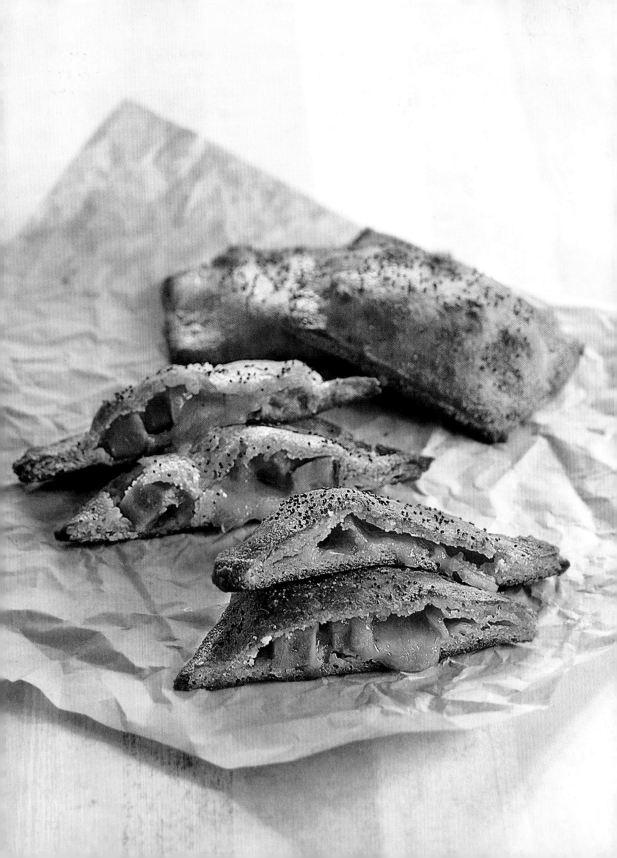

HAM AND CHEESE POCKETS

This recipe is a low-carb twist on a childhood favorite frozen convenience meal. While it requires a little more prep time, it's definitely worth it. These Ham and Cheese Pockets are great for kids because they're handheld and full of cheese, and they have a crispy crust and warm, gooey center!

Prep time 10 minutes | **Cook time** 20 minutes | **Serves 4**

1½ cups shredded mozzarella

2 ounces cream cheese, softened

1 cup finely ground blanched almond flour

1 tablespoon coconut flour

1 teaspoon baking soda

¼ teaspoon apple cider vinegar

1 large egg

4 ounces cooked ham, chopped into cubes

4 ounces sharp Cheddar, shredded

4 teaspoons Dijon mustard

¼ teaspoon poppy seeds

Per Serving

Calories: 543 | Fat: 39g | Protein: 33g | Sodium: 1,373mg | Fiber: 4g | Carbohydrates: 10g | Net Carbohydrates: 6g | Sugar: 3g

1 Preheat the oven to 400°F. Line a large baking sheet with parchment paper.

2 In a large microwave-safe bowl, add mozzarella, cream cheese, almond flour, and coconut flour. Microwave for 45 seconds, then stir. Microwave for an additional 15 seconds and stir until a smooth ball forms.

3 Add baking soda, vinegar, and egg. Stir until combined and a soft ball forms. Separate the dough into four pieces and flatten into 4" × 6" rectangles. Wet your hands with a bit of water to prevent the dough from sticking to your hands as you work, repeating as needed.

4 On one half of each piece of dough, place 1 ounce ham and 1 ounce Cheddar. Fold the other half of the dough over and press to seal it closed.

5 Brush 1 teaspoon mustard over each pocket and sprinkle with poppy seeds and place onto prepared baking sheet. Bake for 15 minutes or until golden brown. Let cool for 10 minutes before serving.

Change Up the Fillings

You can switch up the filling for these pockets however you or your family would like. This cheesy dough can be used with your favorite chopped-up fillings, such as taco meat, turkey, and Cheddar, or even pepperoni! It also makes a great mini calzone—brush the outside with garlic butter and sprinkle with Parmesan before you cook it.

GARLIC BREAD MEATBALL SLIDERS

Garlic bread is the perfect companion for juicy Italian meatballs, and it's made even better when the two are combined! These sliders are a savory, handheld meal filled to the brim with a symphony of perfectly matched flavors. The bread is both cheesy and buttery, which is perfect for the savory meatballs in marinara sauce.

Prep time 10 minutes | **Cook time** 30 minutes | **Serves 8**

2 cups shredded mozzarella

3 tablespoons salted butter, divided

2 cups finely ground blanched almond flour

1½ teaspoons baking powder

1 teaspoon apple cider vinegar

1 medium egg, whisked

¼ teaspoon garlic powder

½ pound 80/20 ground beef

¼ teaspoon dried basil

⅛ teaspoon dried oregano

⅛ teaspoon ground black pepper

¼ teaspoon finely ground pink Himalayan salt

1 tablespoon coconut oil

1 cup low-carb marinara sauce

½ cup grated Parmesan

Per Serving
Calories: 438 | Fat: 33g | Protein: 23g | Sodium: 617mg | Fiber: 3g | Carbohydrates: 10g | Net Carbohydrates: 7g | Sugar: 3g

1 Preheat the oven to 400°F. Line a baking sheet with parchment paper.

2 In a large microwave-safe bowl, add mozzarella, 2 tablespoons butter, and almond flour.

3 Microwave for 45 seconds, then stir. Microwave for an additional 15 seconds, then add baking powder and vinegar. Stir until a soft ball of dough forms.

4 Separate the ball into two even portions, then cut each portion into four. Roll each into a ball, then slightly press down to flatten. Place on the prepared baking sheet. Brush the tops with egg.

5 Bake for 15 minutes or until golden on the bottom and sides. Set aside to cool for at least 15 minutes. In a small bowl, mix the remaining 1 tablespoon butter and garlic powder, then brush over the rolls.

6 In a large bowl, mix ground beef, basil, oregano, and pepper until combined. Form into eight meatballs, about 2 heaping tablespoons of beef per ball. Sprinkle with salt.

7 In a large skillet over medium heat, melt coconut oil. Add the meatballs to the pan and sear, turning to brown each side, about 2 minutes. Reduce the heat to a simmer over low heat, then add marinara sauce to the pan and cover for 7–10 minutes or until the meatballs have an internal temperature of at least 160°F.

8 Slice each roll in half like a bun and place one meatball and 2 tablespoons sauce on each bottom. Sprinkle with 1 tablespoon Parmesan, then place the tops on the sliders and secure with a toothpick, if desired.

90-SECOND BREAD TUNA MELT

This recipe is great when you are short on time but want a home-made meal. This bread cooks up in the microwave quickly, then is toasted for a buttery, crispy outside. If you're not into tuna, don't worry! This bread also tastes great for a grilled cheese sandwich (just add your favorite cheese blend), a burger patty melt, or an egg salad sandwich.

Prep time 2 minutes | **Cook time** 5 minutes | **Serves 1**

2 tablespoons salted butter, divided

4 tablespoons finely ground blanched almond flour

¼ teaspoon baking powder

⅛ teaspoon apple cider vinegar

1 large egg

1 (1-ounce) slice pepper jack

1 (2.6-ounce) pouch tuna

Per Serving

Calories: 592 | Fat: 46g | Protein: 37g | Sodium: 775mg | Fiber: 3g | Carbohydrates: 6g | Net Carbohydrates: 3g | Sugar: 1g

1 In a small microwave-safe bowl, microwave 1 tablespoon butter until melted, about 20 seconds.

2 In a separate small bowl, whisk almond flour and baking powder together. Pour in melted butter and mix. Then stir in vinegar and egg until combined.

3 Transfer the batter into a 4" round microwave-safe glass bowl. Microwave for 90 seconds. Let cool for 2 minutes, then remove the bread from the bowl.

4 Place the remaining 1 tablespoon butter in a small skillet over medium heat. Cut the bread in half, then place half of the cheese slice on the bottom of the bread. Then add tuna and top with the remaining cheese and top of bread.

5 Place the sandwich into the sizzling butter and brown for 2 minutes per side or until golden and crispy. Serve warm.

JICAMA FRIES

If you've never tried jicama, you're in for a treat! It is sweeter and softer than a potato but can have a nice crunch. It's mild and takes on the flavor of your seasoning, and when you bake it, it crisps up like fries! This swap is a little higher in carbs than some other keto options, but it's definitely one of the closest to real potato fries in taste and texture. Serve warm with your favorite low-carb ketchup or high-fat dipping sauce such as ranch.

Prep time 15 minutes | **Cook time** 30 minutes | **Serves 4**

1 medium jicama, peeled and sliced (1"-wide and ¼"-thick fries)

3 tablespoons olive oil

½ teaspoon paprika

¼ teaspoon sea salt

⅛ teaspoon ground black pepper

Per Serving
Calories: 137 | Fat: 8g | Protein: 1g | Sodium: 104mg | Fiber: 8g | Carbohydrates: 15g | Net Carbohydrates: 7g | Sugar: 3g

1 Preheat the oven to 400°F.

2 In a medium pot over medium-high heat, boil 6 cups water. Once water begins to boil, add jicama. Reduce the temperature to medium and cook for 10 minutes.

3 Remove the fries from the water and place on a kitchen towel. Pat completely dry, using a second towel if necessary. Drizzle with olive oil and sprinkle with paprika, salt, and pepper.

4 Bake for 20 minutes, flipping halfway through. When done, fries will be golden and crispy. Serve warm.

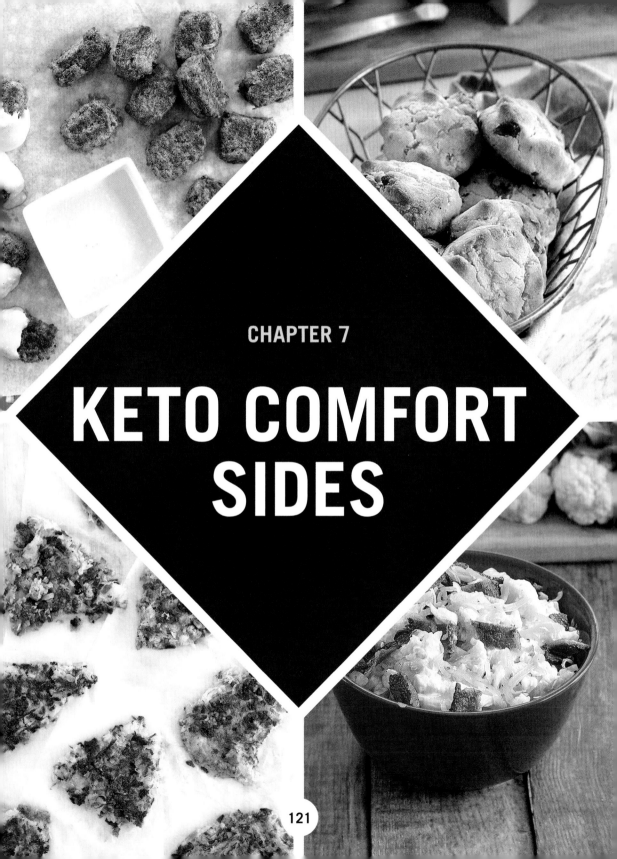

CHAPTER 7

KETO COMFORT SIDES

ZUCCHINI CHIPS

These chips make the perfect dipper for all your favorite high-fat sauces like ranch and queso! The trick to making these extracrispy is removing all the excess moisture. That will leave them with a milder taste that can be easily adapted to your favorite flavors.

Prep time 60 minutes | **Cook time** 60 minutes | **Serves 4**

4 medium zucchini
½ teaspoon finely ground sea salt

Per Serving
Calories: 33 | Fat: 0g | Protein: 2g | Sodium: 210mg | Fiber: 2g | Carbohydrates: 6g | Net Carbohydrates: 4g | Sugar: 4g

1 Use a mandoline to slice zucchini into ¼" uniform slices. Place the slices on paper towels or a kitchen towel and sprinkle with salt. Place another two layers of paper towels on top of the slices and put a cast-iron pan or other weighted item on top. Let the water absorb for 1 hour.

2 Preheat the oven to 300°F. Line two large baking sheets with parchment paper. Place the zucchini slices onto the sheet and bake for 1 hour or until golden and crispy. For best freshness, store in an airtight container at room temperature for up to 4 days.

MASHED CAULIFLOWER AND GRAVY

Potatoes are one of the ultimate comfort foods because of their versatility. Cauliflower may taste a bit different, but it's incredibly adaptable, and with the right seasoning, it can give you wonderful, comforting feelings too. The cream cheese helps give it a smooth texture closer to real potatoes, and the sour cream brightens it and adds flavor. Once you add the gravy, you might be surprised that the carb lovers in your family prefer this!

Prep time 5 minutes | **Cook time** 20 minutes | **Serves 4**

1 medium head cauliflower, leaves removed, cored, and cut into florets

4 tablespoons salted butter, cubed

⅛ teaspoon finely ground pink Himalayan salt

⅛ teaspoon ground black pepper

¼ cup sour cream

2 ounces cream cheese

2 tablespoons unsalted butter

1 cup chicken bone broth

⅓ cup heavy whipping cream

¼ teaspoon xanthan gum

Per Serving
Calories: 347 | Fat: 30g | Protein: 7g | Sodium: 311mg | Fiber: 3g | Carbohydrates: 9g | Net Carbohydrates: 6g | Sugar: 4g

1 Pour 2 cups water into a large pot over medium-high heat and bring it to a boil. Place a steamer basket into the pot and add cauliflower.

2 Cover and let steam for 10 minutes until fork-tender. Carefully remove the steamer basket and place cauliflower into a food processor.

3 Place salted butter, salt, pepper, sour cream, and cream cheese into the food processor. Turn it on low for 30–45 seconds or until the mixture is smooth. (Feel free to leave it a little chunky if that is your preference.)

4 To prepare the gravy, place unsalted butter, chicken bone broth, and heavy whipping cream in a small saucepan and whisk over medium heat until the mixture is reduced by about a third, about 5 minutes, then whisk in xanthan gum. Turn off the heat and allow the gravy to thicken for 3 minutes, whisking occasionally. Pour the gravy over scoops of mashed cauliflower to serve.

"FAUXTATO" SALAD

What's a summer barbecue without a bowl of potato salad? This recipe will give you all the best flavor and textures of a real potato salad with just a fraction of the carbs. The tangy cream sauce combined with a fresh crunch from the green onion will pair with all your favorite barbecue main dishes and have your guests asking for more. This is also a great recipe for those picky eaters who don't like cauliflower—you can't even taste that it's in here!

Prep time 10 minutes | **Cook time** 10 minutes | **Serves 6**

1 large head cauliflower, leaves removed, cored, stems removed, and tops cut into bite-sized pieces

½ cup mayonnaise

2 teaspoons yellow mustard

1 tablespoon dill pickle relish

4 slices cooked bacon, chopped

½ cup shredded mild Cheddar

2 medium stalks green onion, sliced

Per Serving
Calories: 238 | Fat: 19g | Protein: 8g | Sodium: 393mg | Fiber: 3g | Carbohydrates: 8g | Net Carbohydrates: 5g | Sugar: 3g

1 Pour 2 cups water into a medium pot over medium heat and place a steamer basket into the water.

2 Carefully place cauliflower into the basket and cover. Allow to steam for 7 minutes or until cauliflower is fork-tender but not mushy.

3 Remove cauliflower and place into a large bowl of cold water.

4 In a separate large bowl, mix mayonnaise, mustard, and relish. Add the cold cauliflower to the bowl and fold into the wet mixture.

5 Sprinkle with bacon and Cheddar. Garnish with green onion. Serve cold.

Short on Time?

If you're short on time, feel free to use a steamer bag of cauliflower! Two 12-ounce bags of cauliflower will give you the perfect amount and make this recipe even easier. Feel free to prep this recipe the day before you plan to eat it to allow the flavors time to meld.

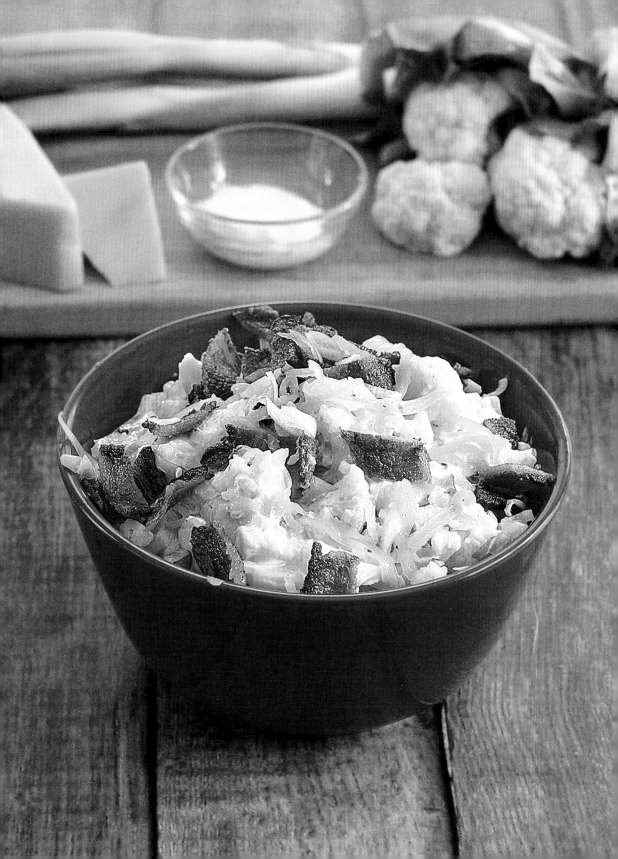

SKILLET "CORN" BREAD

Nothing warms you up like a hot bowl of chili and a buttery slice of corn bread. While this recipe contains no cornmeal, you'll find that almond flour gives you a similar texture. This dish has just a hint of sweetness that will complement a spicy dish.

Prep time 10 minutes | **Cook time** 15 minutes | **Serves 6**

1¼ cups finely ground blanched almond flour

2 teaspoons baking powder

1 teaspoon granular erythritol

¼ cup sour cream

2 ounces cream cheese, softened

4 tablespoons salted butter, melted

⅛ teaspoon finely ground pink Himalayan salt

3 large eggs

1 Preheat the oven to 400°F.

2 In a large bowl, mix all the ingredients. Pour into a 6" cast-iron skillet or other similarly sized oven-safe pan.

3 Bake for 15 minutes or until edges are golden and a toothpick inserted in the center comes out clean. Cool for 15 minutes before serving.

Per Serving
Calories: 298 | Fat: 26g | Protein: 9g | Sodium: 330mg | Fiber: 3g | Carbohydrates: 6g | Sugar Alcohol: 1g | Net Carbohydrates: 3g | Sugar: 2g

Spice It Up

If you love spicy things, you can turn this into cheesy jalapeño bread! Add 1 cup Cheddar and ¼ cup chopped pickled jalapeños for a fun twist. This recipe would also pair great with Spicy White Chicken Chili (see recipe in Chapter 3) or Pickle-Brined Crispy Chicken (see recipe in Chapter 6).

SAUSAGE "CORN" BREAD STUFFING

Nothing says holiday comfort food quite like stuffing. This version includes pork, which adds extra fat. The seasoning kicks it up a notch to make it truly a side to remember while keeping you on track with your keto goals. The recipe requires making the corn bread first, so be sure you plan ahead for the extra time.

Prep time 20 minutes | **Cook time** 45 minutes | **Serves 8**

½ pound ground pork sausage
¼ medium yellow onion, peeled and diced
1 medium stalk celery, chopped
¼ cup chicken broth
⅛ teaspoon ground black pepper
⅛ teaspoon dried sage
⅛ teaspoon dried rosemary
1 large egg
2 tablespoons heavy whipping cream
1 recipe Skillet "Corn" Bread (see recipe in this chapter)

Per Serving
Calories: 347 | Fat: 27g | Protein: 14g | Sodium: 481mg | Fiber: 1g | Carbohydrates: 9g | Net Carbohydrates: 8g | Sugar: 2g

1 Preheat the oven to 400°F.

2 In a medium skillet over medium heat, brown sausage until no pink remains, about 12 minutes. Add onion and celery to the pan and cook for an additional 4–5 minutes or until celery softens.

3 Pour the mixture into a large bowl and add broth, pepper, sage, and rosemary. Whisk in egg and heavy whipping cream.

4 Break cooled Skillet "Corn" Bread into bite-sized pieces and gently toss with the other ingredients until all pieces are coated.

5 Transfer the bowl contents into an 8" × 8" baking dish. Bake for 25 minutes or until the top and edges are golden brown. Let cool for 10 minutes before serving.

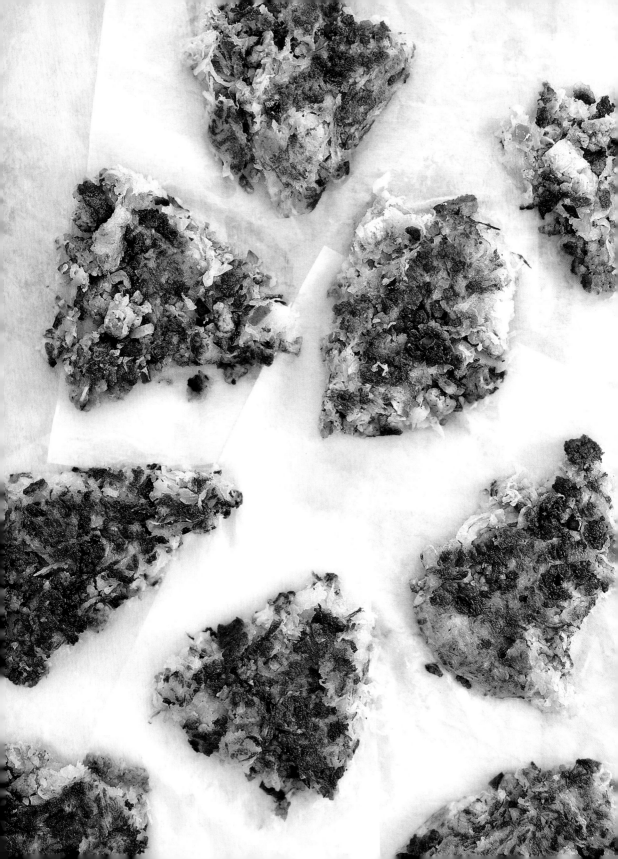

SAUSAGE AND JICAMA HASH

This dish is a great alternative when you want something for breakfast that isn't eggs. While eggs are delicious, they tend to be the primary go-to ingredient for ketogenic breakfasts. This recipe uses jicama, which, when grated, has a texture similar to potatoes. The peppers and onions will remind you of the classic O'Brien potatoes dish but with way fewer carbs.

Prep time 15 minutes | **Cook time** 25 minutes | **Serves 6**

1 (2-pound) jicama, peeled and grated

1 pound pork breakfast sausage

¼ medium yellow onion, peeled and diced

½ medium green bell pepper, seeded and diced

2 tablespoons coconut oil

Per Serving

Calories: 299 | Fat: 20g | Protein: 13g | Sodium: 735mg | Fiber: 7g | Carbohydrates: 15g | Net Carbohydrates: 8g | Sugar: 3g

1 Place grated jicama into a kitchen towel and remove as much moisture as possible, then set aside.

2 In a medium skillet over medium heat, cook sausage until no pink remains, about 12 minutes. Drain the excess grease from the pan and add onion, bell pepper, coconut oil, and jicama to the pan.

3 Let the ingredients cook for about 5 minutes until crispy, then flip and cook for an additional 5 minutes until brown and crispy. Serve warm.

SQUASH AU GRATIN

This is a creamy dish that is great for getting the family involved. Once you've sliced the summer squash and zucchini, let the kids have fun arranging the slices into layers while you whip up the creamy sauce. In just minutes, you'll have it in the oven, and you'll love knowing that you made it together.

Prep time 5 minutes | **Cook time** 30 minutes | **Serves 4**

2 medium yellow summer squash, sliced

2 medium zucchini, sliced

4 tablespoons salted butter

¼ medium yellow onion, peeled and diced

2 ounces cream cheese, softened

½ cup heavy whipping cream

¼ cup vegetable broth

¼ teaspoon xanthan gum

½ cup grated Parmesan

⅛ teaspoon ground black pepper

⅛ teaspoon finely ground sea salt

2 ounces plain pork rinds, finely ground

Per Serving
Calories: 422 | Fat: 34g | Protein: 16g | Sodium: 705mg | Fiber: 3g | Carbohydrates: 11g | Net Carbohydrates: 8g | Sugar: 6g

1 Preheat the oven to 400°F. Place the sliced squash and zucchini between two kitchen towels to absorb excess moisture.

2 In a medium skillet over medium heat, melt butter. Add onion and sauté 3 minutes until it begins to soften. Whisk in cream cheese, heavy whipping cream, vegetable broth, and xanthan gum. Allow to come to a boil, then reduce heat to low heat to a simmer, whisking occasionally for 3 minutes. The sauce will reduce and thicken.

3 Sprinkle in Parmesan, pepper, and salt. Place squash and zucchini into a 4-quart baking dish in layers as necessary. Pour the cream sauce over the vegetables. Sprinkle pork rinds on top and bake for 20 minutes or until bubbling and golden. Let cool for 10 minutes before serving.

LOADED CAULIFLOWER

This dish is the perfect complement to any main dish and is tasty on its own as well. The cheese gives it a creamy texture that, when paired with crispy bacon and fresh onion, is reminiscent of a loaded baked potato. You can even add your own shredded meat, such as pulled pork, into the dish for a complete meal!

Prep time 10 minutes | **Cook time** 5 minutes | **Serves 4**

1 (12-ounce) steamer bag cauliflower florets

4 ounces cream cheese, softened

2 tablespoons sour cream

¼ teaspoon finely ground pink Himalayan salt

¼ teaspoon garlic powder

¼ teaspoon ground black pepper

1 cup shredded sharp Cheddar

6 slices cooked bacon, crumbled

1 medium stalk green onion, sliced

Per Serving
Calories: 325 | Fat: 24g | Protein: 16g | Sodium: 696mg | Fiber: 2g | Carbohydrates: 6g | Net Carbohydrates: 4g | Sugar: 3g

1 Cook cauliflower according to package instructions, about 5 minutes, then place in a food processor. Add cream cheese and sour cream and pulse until almost smooth, while a few chunks remain (about ten pulses).

2 Transfer the mixture to a large bowl and fold in salt, garlic powder, and pepper. Smooth the top layer. Top with Cheddar, bacon, and green onion. Serve warm.

EASY CHEESE BREAD

This is one of the best recipes for kids and keto newbies because everyone can get involved in prep and it takes no time at all. It's a one-bowl wonder that comes together in a snap.

Prep time 5 minutes | **Cook time** 20 minutes | **Serves 6**

1 cup shredded mozzarella
¼ cup shredded sharp Cheddar
1 large egg
¼ teaspoon garlic powder
¼ teaspoon dried basil
¼ teaspoon dried oregano

Per Serving
Calories: 84 | Fat: 6g | Protein: 7g | Sodium: 142mg | Fiber: 0g | Carbohydrates: 1g | Net Carbohydrates: 1g | Sugar: 0g

1 Preheat the oven to 400°F. Line a large baking sheet with parchment paper.

2 In a large bowl, mix all the ingredients until fully combined.

3 Scoop the mixture into the center of the prepared baking sheet. Wet your hands with water, then firmly press down the mixture to form an 8" × 8" square. Bake for 20 minutes or until golden and bubbling.

4 Let cool for 10 minutes, then cut into 6 slices. Serve warm.

Customize It!

This bread is a great canvas for your favorite pizza toppings! Simply mix in your favorite meat, and/or vegetables or even swap out the cheese for a different variety. The great thing about this recipe, besides how simple it is, is how versatile it is. You can even top it with pizza sauce so it becomes a crust.

CHORIZO QUESO

If you love gooey, cheesy restaurant-style queso, you have to try this keto-friendly version. It includes spicy chorizo and comes together in less than 20 minutes! It's perfect for movie night or even just as a meal paired with pork rinds, cheese crisps, and vegetables for dipping.

Prep time 5 minutes | **Cook time** 15 minutes | **Yields 2 cups, ¼ cup per serving**

¼ pound ground Mexican chorizo
¼ cup salted butter
¼ medium yellow onion, peeled and chopped
3 ounces cream cheese, softened
½ cup heavy whipping cream
¼ cup chicken broth
8 ounces white American cheese, cubed

Per Serving
Calories: 272 | Fat: 23g | Protein: 9g | Sodium: 675mg | Fiber: 0g | Carbohydrates: 5g | Net Carbohydrates: 5g | Sugar: 3g

1 In a medium saucepan over medium heat, cook chorizo, about 7 minutes. Drain the grease and set chorizo aside in a small bowl.

2 Return the pan to the stovetop and melt butter. Sauté onion for 3 minutes until fragrant. Whisk in cream cheese, heavy whipping cream, and broth. Simmer for 3 minutes, then whisk in white American cheese until completely smooth, about 1 minute.

3 Add the cooked chorizo to the pan and fold in until combined. Serve warm.

Make It Your Own!

If you're not a fan of chorizo, feel free to swap for taco-seasoned ground beef or chicken. You can also use a can of drained diced tomatoes and chilies. Get creative and see what unique creations you can come up with!

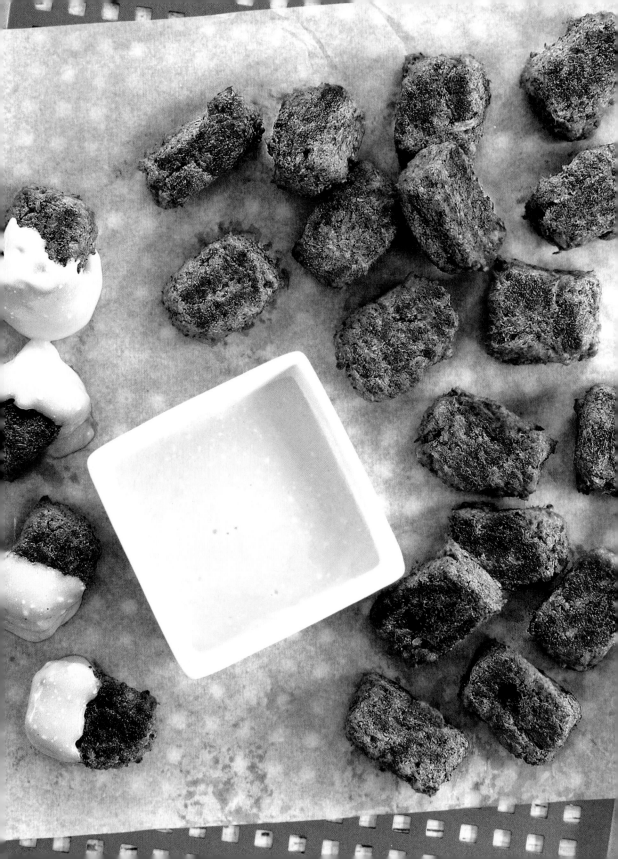

CHEESY BROCCOLI TOTS

Tater Tots are always a comfort food. They're crispy, they're quick, and everyone likes them. Most keto swaps call for cauliflower instead of potatoes, but if you're feeling a bit tired of cauliflower, this recipe is for you! The broccoli is a nice alternative because it's full of nutrients and still very dippable. Try it with your favorite cheese sauce for dipping!

Prep time 10 minutes | **Cook time** 20 minutes | **Serves 5**

2 (12-ounce) steamer bags broccoli florets

2 ounces cream cheese, softened

1 cup shredded Cheddar

2 ounces 100% Parmesan cheese crisps, finely ground

1 egg

Per Serving

Calories: 211 | Fat: 13g | Protein: 14g | Sodium: 372mg | Fiber: 4g | Carbohydrates: 8g | Net Carbohydrates: 4g | Sugar: 2g

1 Preheat the oven to 400°F. Line a baking sheet with parchment paper.

2 Cook broccoli according to package instructions. Drain the excess moisture from broccoli in a kitchen towel, then place broccoli into a food processor. Add the remaining ingredients to the food processor and pulse until smooth, about twenty pulses. Scrape down the sides as needed.

3 Let the mixture sit for 5 minutes, then scoop 2 table-spoons of it and roll into a Tater Tot shape. Repeat with the remaining mixture to form twenty pieces and place on the prepared baking sheet.

4 Bake for 15 minutes, flipping halfway through the cook time. The broccoli pieces will be golden and firm when done. Let cool for 10 minutes before serving.

Cheese Dipping Sauce

To make a quick cheese sauce, melt 2 tablespoons butter, then whisk in 2 ounces cream cheese and ½ cup heavy whipping cream. Once that starts bubbling, about 3 minutes, add in 1 cup fresh shredded Cheddar and whisk until smooth. It's as easy as that!

COLESLAW

Coleslaw is a classic side for everything from grilled fish to grilled chicken, but traditional coleslaw recipes can carry as many as 30 grams of carbs per serving! That's because the sauce is typically loaded with sugar to give it that familiar sweet flavor. Say good-bye to the unnecessary sugar with this recipe, and be sure to pack it along for your next barbecue.

Prep time 5 minutes | **Cook time** N/A | **Serves 4**

½ cup mayonnaise

¼ cup sour cream

1 teaspoon powdered erythritol

2 tablespoons apple cider vinegar

4 cups shredded green cabbage

Per Serving
Calories: 233 | Fat: 37g | Protein: 1g | Sodium: 194mg | Fiber: 2g | Carbohydrates: 5g | Sugar Alcohol: 1g | Net Carbohydrates: 3g | Sugar: 3g

In a large bowl, whisk mayonnaise, sour cream, erythritol, and vinegar. Fold in cabbage and cover with plastic wrap. Let sit for at least 30 minutes in the refrigerator. Serve chilled.

Add Some Spice

Add 2 tablespoons chopped pickled jalapeño and juice from half a lime to spice up this recipe. It will be a sweet, tart, and spicy taste that will go great with just about any grilled protein—perfect for summer!

GREEN BEAN CASSEROLE

This comfort classic just got even better! Traditionally, this dish uses canned soup, which has a lot of carbs and preservatives. Luckily, it's supereasy to make a sauce that's just as tasty! This sauce is creamy and has bits of mushrooms, just like the condensed soup.

Prep time 10 minutes | **Cook time** 35 minutes | **Serves 6**

1 pound green beans, trimmed

2 tablespoons salted butter

½ cup cremini mushrooms, chopped

1 clove garlic, peeled and minced

3 ounces cream cheese, softened

½ cup heavy whipping cream

½ cup chicken broth

¼ teaspoon finely ground pink Himalayan salt

⅛ teaspoon ground black pepper

¼ teaspoon xanthan gum

2 ounces 100% Parmesan cheese crisps, crushed

Per Serving
Calories: 197 | Fat: 17g | Protein: 5g | Sodium: 513mg | Fiber: 2g | Carbohydrates: 5g | Net Carbohydrates: 3g | Sugar: 2g

1 Preheat the oven to 400°F.

2 Pour 2 cups water into a large pot over medium-high heat. Place a steamer basket into the bottom of the pot. Cut green beans into bite-sized pieces. Once the water is boiling, carefully place green beans into the steamer basket. Cover and let steam for 5 minutes.

3 In a medium saucepan over medium heat, melt butter. Sauté mushrooms until they begin to soften, about 3 minutes. Add garlic and sauté for 30 seconds.

4 Whisk in cream cheese, heavy whipping cream, broth, salt, pepper, and xanthan gum. Reduce the heat to a low simmer and continue to cook for 4 minutes or until the mixture begins to thicken, whisking frequently.

5 Carefully remove the steamer basket and place green beans into an 8" × 8" casserole dish. Pour the sauce into the pan and carefully fold green beans into the sauce. Top with cheese crisps. Bake for 20 minutes until bubbling. Let cool for 10 minutes, then serve warm.

Legumes

While some may choose to avoid legumes while following a ketogenic diet, others may feel they're fine to incorporate. Ultimately, the decision is up to you. It's always important to do your own research and decide how you want your personal journey to look.

CHEDDAR BACON BISCUITS

These savory biscuits are the perfect bread-like side to complement your entrée! The sour cream helps keep them moist while baking so you don't end up with a mouthful of dry biscuit. You can also slice these in half to use as keto sandwich buns.

Prep time 5 minutes | **Cook time** 15 minutes | **Serves 8**

2 cups finely ground blanched almond flour

2 teaspoons baking powder

¼ teaspoon baking soda

4 tablespoons cold salted butter

⅓ cup sour cream

1 large egg

½ teaspoon apple cider vinegar

½ cup shredded sharp Cheddar

3 slices cooked bacon, crumbled

Per Serving
Calories: 287 | Fat: 21g | Protein: 12g | Sodium: 338mg | Fiber: 2g | Carbohydrates: 11g | Net Carbohydrates: 9g | Sugar: 2g

1 Preheat the oven to 350°F. Line a large baking sheet with parchment paper.

2 Place almond flour, baking powder, and baking soda in a food processor. Pulse a few times to combine. Add butter and sour cream, then pulse until combined, about five times.

3 Turn the food processor on low and then crack open egg into the processor and pour in vinegar. Pulse three to five times to combine. Remove the food processor blade, then fold in Cheddar and bacon. Let the dough rest for 5 minutes.

4 Spoon about 3 tablespoons of dough onto the prepared baking sheet. Then repeat with the remaining dough to make eight biscuits, leaving at least 2"of space in between.

5 Bake for 12–14 minutes or until edges are golden and a toothpick inserted in the center comes out clean. Let cool for at least 15 minutes before serving. Store in an airtight container in the refrigerator up to 4 days for best freshness.

Why Vinegar?

Vinegar helps make keto baked goods fluffy. Baking soda and baking powder on their own do cause keto-friendly flour to rise, but adding in a little vinegar will create a better rise and help the dough hold together. Plus, you won't even be able to taste it!

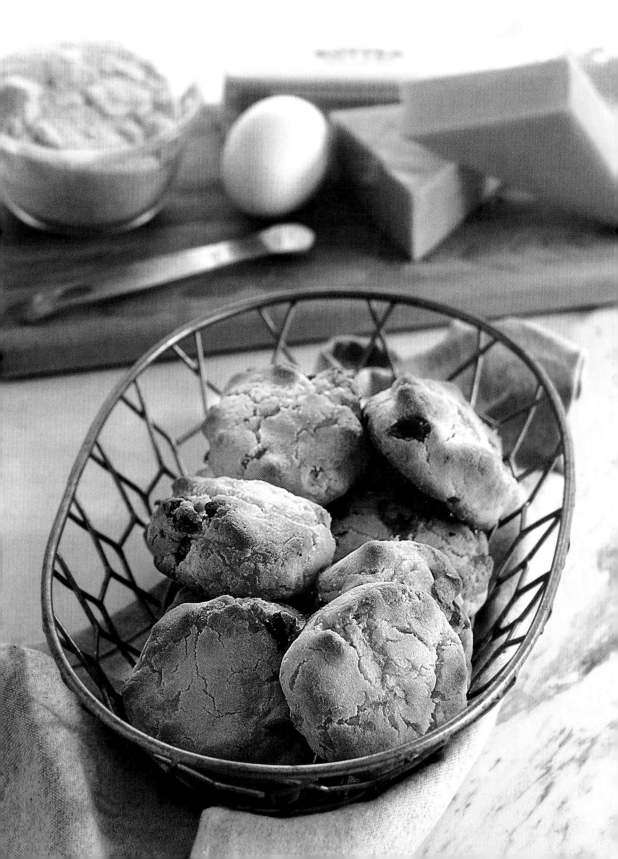

CREAMED SPINACH

Although ketogenic macronutrients are most frequently discussed, the micronutrients are important too! This cheesy dish will surprise even those picky eaters. A big bowl of spinach can feel a little overwhelming, but with this dish you'll be amazed at how much it cooks down.

Prep time 5 minutes | **Cook time** 15 minutes | **Serves 4**

2 tablespoons salted butter

¼ medium white onion, peeled and diced

1 clove garlic, peeled and minced

1 pound fresh spinach, ends trimmed

2 ounces cream cheese, softened

¼ cup chicken broth

¼ cup heavy whipping cream

¼ cup grated Parmesan

1 In a large skillet over medium heat, melt butter. Sauté onion for 3 minutes until it begins to soften.

2 Add garlic and spinach to the pan and sauté for 1 minute, then add cream cheese then pour in broth and heavy whipping cream. Reduce heat to low and simmer; continue stirring and letting the moisture evaporate until it becomes thick and creamy, about 7 minutes.

3 Sprinkle in Parmesan and serve warm.

Per Serving
Calories: 207 | Fat: 17g | Protein: 6g | Sodium: 362mg | Fiber: 3g | Carbohydrates: 7g | Net Carbohydrates: 4g | Sugar: 2g

Spinach Is a Superfood!

Spinach is one of the healthiest vegetables out there. Not only is it packed with essential vitamins and minerals (like calcium), but it's also a great source of fiber, which can aid in weight loss.

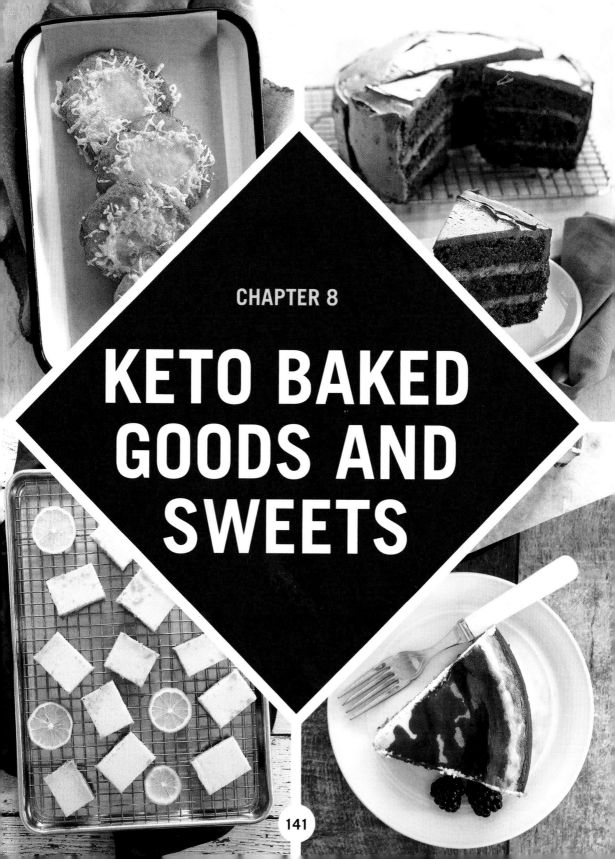

CHAPTER 8

KETO BAKED GOODS AND SWEETS

EASY FUDGE

This chocolaty dessert is dense and decadent, and even better, it's extremely simple to make. Thanks to the secret ingredient of keto-friendly sweetened condensed milk (made with whipping cream, butter, and erythritol), it keeps its shape and won't melt in your hands like many high-fat fudges! Make sure the chocolate chips you use are actually low-carb, not just sugar-free. (Some brands use sweeteners like maltitol, which are actually high glycemic and can cause digestive troubles.) Instead, look for chocolate chips that use natural sweeteners like stevia.

Prep time 5 minutes | **Cook time** 20 minutes | **Serves 12**

1 cup heavy whipping cream
⅓ cup powdered erythritol
2 tablespoons unsalted butter
1 teaspoon vanilla extract
1 cup low-carb chocolate chips
¼ cup chopped pecans

Per Serving
Calories: 168 | Fat: 16g |
Protein: 2g | Sodium: 22mg |
Fiber: 6g | Carbohydrates: 17g |
Sugar Alcohol: 8g |
Net Carbohydrates: 7g | Sugar: 1g

1 In a small saucepan over medium heat, mix heavy whipping cream, erythritol, butter, and vanilla. Stir often and scrape the sides down, for about 20 minutes, until golden brown, thick, sweetened condensed milk forms.

2 Remove from heat and let cool for 15 minutes before stirring in chocolate chips.

3 Line a 9" × 5" loaf pan with parchment paper. Once chocolate chips are melted, pour the mixture into the prepared pan. Top with pecans before cooling in refrigerator for at least 1 hour. Slice into twelve bars and serve chilled. Store in an airtight container in the refrigerator up to 4 days for best taste.

No Chocolate Chips? No Problem!

If you don't have sugar-free chocolate chips on hand, you can add ⅓ cup unsweetened cocoa powder to the completely cooled (that's important) sweetened condensed milk that forms. If you go this route, you'll want to taste the mix as you go in case you need to add extra powdered erythritol to match your preferred sweetness.

BANANA BREAD

With 27 grams of carbs in a medium banana, the fruit itself isn't the best option for a keto diet. This recipe uses banana extract to replicate the classic banana bread you ate for breakfast as a child, with just a fraction of the carbs. Go ahead, cut yourself a second slice!

Prep time 10 minutes | **Cook time** 25 minutes | **Serves 12**

1½ cups plus 1 tablespoon finely ground blanched almond flour, divided

½ cup plus 1 tablespoon granular erythritol, divided

2 tablespoons ground golden flax

2 teaspoons baking powder

½ teaspoon ground cinnamon

4 tablespoons unsalted butter, melted

2½ teaspoons banana extract

1 teaspoon vanilla extract

¼ cup unsweetened almond milk

¼ cup sour cream

2 large eggs

¾ cup chopped walnuts

1 tablespoon cold salted butter

Per Serving
Calories: 210 | Fat: 19g | Protein: 6g | Sodium: 107mg | Fiber: 2g | Carbohydrates: 14g | Sugar Alcohol: 9g | Net Carbohydrates: 8g | Sugar: 2g

1 Preheat the oven to 350°F.

2 In a large bowl, mix 1½ cups almond flour, ½ cup erythritol, flax, baking powder, and cinnamon.

3 Pour in melted butter, then add banana extract, vanilla, almond milk, sour cream, and eggs. Mix until combined.

4 Pour the batter into a nonstick 9" × 5" loaf pan.

5 Place walnuts, salted butter, the remaining almond flour, and the remaining erythritol in a food processor and pulse five times to make a crumble. Sprinkle over the top of the loaf, then place into the oven to bake for 25 minutes. Allow to cool for 30 minutes before removing from the pan and then completely cool to avoid crumbling.

Using Banana Extract

Banana extract is the best way to achieve banana flavoring on a keto diet. It can be found in most grocery stores, but it's also available to order online. This recipe uses a larger amount of extract than you may be used to, but it's necessary to create that comforting banana flavor without using any bananas.

BLACKBERRY DRIZZLE CHEESECAKE

What can beat a sweet and creamy cheesecake for dessert? This fruity creation uses pecans and almond flour to make a decadent crust that rivals any of the high-carb graham cracker crusts you may be used to. If blackberries aren't your favorite, feel free to substitute another low-carb berry, like strawberries. At only about 8 grams of net carbs per cup, they're an excellent alternative. This recipe requires an overnight cooling for best results.

Prep time overnight | **Cook time** 75 minutes | **Serves 16**

1¾ cups whole pecans

3 tablespoons unsalted butter

¼ cup finely ground blanched almond flour

32 ounces cream cheese, softened

1¼ cups powdered erythritol

½ cup sour cream

1 tablespoon vanilla extract

3 large eggs

2 cups blackberries

3 tablespoons water

2 tablespoons granular erythritol

1 Preheat the oven to 350°F.

2 Place pecans, butter, and almond flour into a food processor and pulse until it is the texture of wet sand, about ten pulses, scraping down the sides with a rubber spatula as needed.

3 Press the mixture firmly into a 9" round springform pan and bake for 12 minutes until golden. Set aside to cool for at least 15 minutes.

4 In a large bowl, stir cream cheese with a wooden spoon until it is creamy and smooth. There should be no lumps in cream cheese. Add powdered erythritol and slowly mix until smooth.

5 Stir in sour cream and vanilla. The mixture should still be as smooth as possible. If there are lumps in the batter, there will be lumps in the cheesecake.

6 Add eggs, gently stirring in one at a time. Don't rush this part—overbeating causes air bubbles and will make the cheesecake brown in the oven too quickly.

7 Pour the batter into the cooled crust. Gently tap it against the counter to remove any air bubbles. Bake for 50 minutes. Check after 25 minutes and again at 40 minutes to avoid overcooking due to oven hot spots, gently turning as needed. When done, the center should be slightly jiggly and the edges mostly set. Residual heat will finish the cooking process.

continued . . .

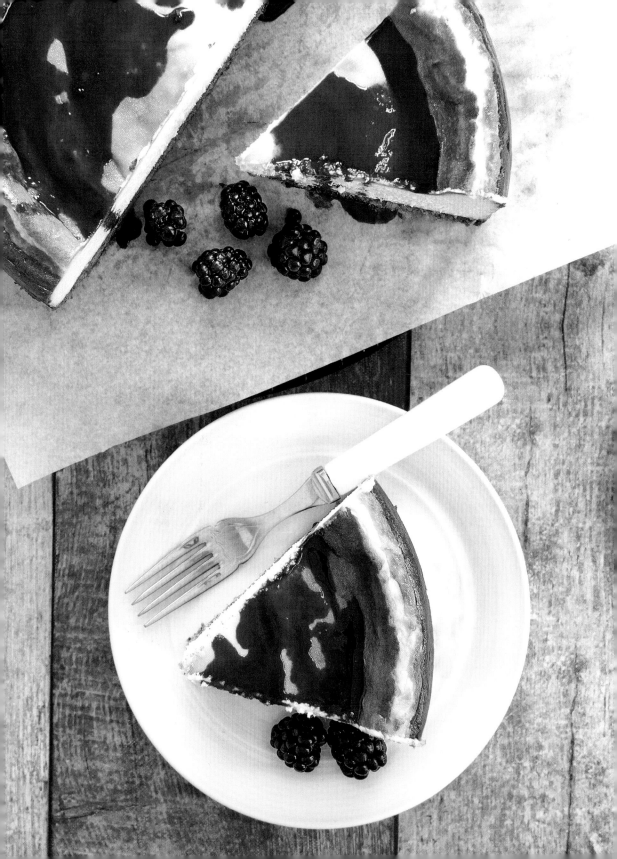

BLACKBERRY DRIZZLE CHEESECAKE (CONTINUED)

Per Serving
Calories: 335 | Fat: 29g | Protein: 6g | Sodium: 224mg | Fiber: 2g | Carbohydrates: 19g | Sugar Alcohol: 13g | Net Carbohydrates: 11g | Sugar: 4g

8 Let cool for 2 hours at room temperature, then place in the refrigerator overnight.

9 To make the blackberry sauce, place blackberries, water, and granular erythritol in a small saucepan over low heat. Allow the mixture to simmer for 10 minutes, then strain the seeds and return the sauce back to the stove to reduce for an additional 2–3 minutes. Remove from the heat and place the mixture in a small bowl to cool.

10 To serve, slice into sixteen pieces and drizzle with 1 tablespoon blackberry sauce.

Avoid Overmixing!

Be careful not to overmix the cheesecake batter. Overmixing can happen easily and leave you with air bubbles that prevent a dense and creamy cheesecake. Extra air also makes the cheesecake brown faster in the oven. An easy way to avoid mixing it too much is to stir by hand, not using a mixer. It may take a bit longer, but the added caution is worth it!

BLUEBERRY MUFFINS

Get ready to start your day off right as you welcome this recipe into your routine! These fresh and fluffy Blueberry Muffins allow you to re-create the goodness of the classic bakery treat at home, low-carb style. Blueberries aren't the lowest-carb berry, but they're okay to enjoy in moderation. Feel free to swap with blackberries, which are lower in carbs, if that better fits your nutritional needs.

Prep time 10 minutes | **Cook time** 20 minutes | **Serves 6**

1 cup finely ground blanched almond flour

2 teaspoons baking powder

¾ cup unsweetened almond milk

2 teaspoons vanilla extract

1 large egg

¼ cup sour cream

4 tablespoons unsalted butter, melted

½ cup granular erythritol

2 teaspoons lemon juice

1 teaspoon apple cider vinegar

⅓ cup coconut flour

½ cup blueberries

4 tablespoons salted cold butter

½ cup chopped pecans

⅛ teaspoon ground cinnamon

Per Serving
Calories: 379 | Fat: 35g | Protein: 7g | Sodium: 275mg | Fiber: 4g | Carbohydrates: 26g | Sugar Alcohol: 16g | Net Carbohydrates: 14g | Sugar: 5g

1 Preheat the oven to 350°F.

2 In a large bowl, mix almond flour and baking powder. Whisk in almond milk, vanilla, egg, sour cream, unsalted butter, erythritol, lemon juice, and apple cider vinegar until well combined.

3 In a medium bowl, toss coconut flour and blueberries, add to the batter and fold in until just mixed.

4 Pour the batter into six paper-lined muffin cups.

5 Place salted butter, pecans, and cinnamon in a food processor and pulse until a crumbly mixture forms, about 30 seconds. Top each muffin with 1 tablespoon of the mixture. Bake for 18 minutes or until edges are golden.

6 Let cool completely before serving. Store in an airtight container in the refrigerator up to 3 days for best freshness.

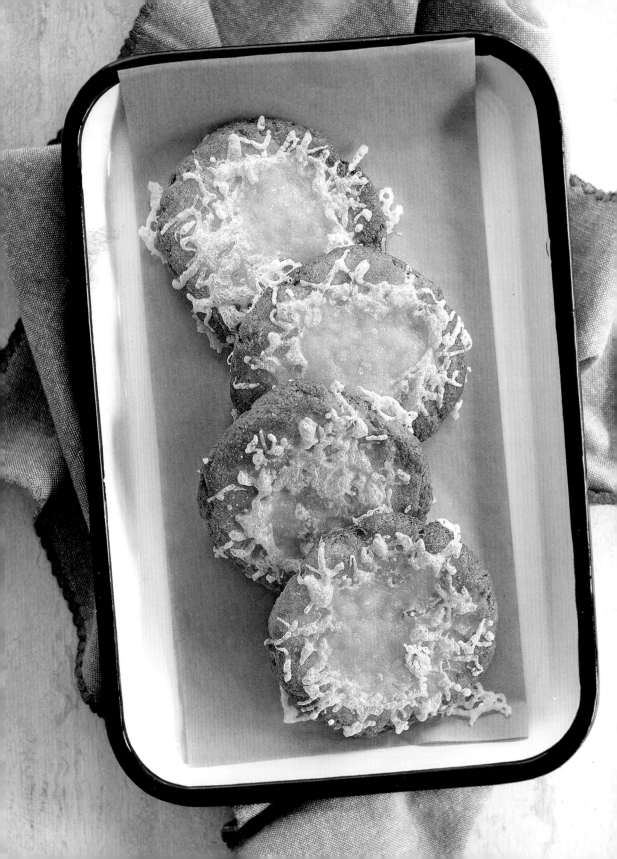

ASIAGO BAGELS

If you're a fan of Asiago Bagels, you know that there's something special about that cheese, and thankfully you don't have to be separated from your breakfast love any longer with this easy-to-bake recipe. Feel free to enjoy these with cream cheese or build them up into the ultimate breakfast sandwich with sausage and cheese.

Prep time 10 minutes | **Cook time** 20 minutes | **Serves 4**

1 cup finely ground blanched almond flour
1½ cups shredded mozzarella
3 tablespoons salted butter
½ teaspoon baking powder
2 large egg whites
3 ounces shredded Asiago

Per Serving
Calories: 467 | Fat: 37g | Protein: 23g | Sodium: 700mg | Fiber: 3g | Carbohydrates: 8g | Net Carbohydrates: 5g | Sugar: 2g

1 Preheat the oven to 400°F. Line a baking sheet with parchment paper.

2 In a large microwave-safe bowl, mix almond flour, mozzarella, butter, and baking powder.

3 Microwave the mixture for 90 seconds or until mozzarella and butter melt together. Stir the mixture with a rubber spatula until a soft dough forms.

4 Add egg whites to the mixture and stir until well combined. The dough will be mostly smooth and very soft but not wet.

5 With wet hands, separate the dough into four even balls. Place the balls onto the prepared baking sheet and flatten slightly to form discs.

6 Bake for 15 minutes. At the 10-minute mark, remove the bagels and sprinkle with Asiago cheese before returning to the oven for 5 more minutes. Allow to cool for 30 minutes before removing from the pan and serving. Store leftovers in an airtight container in the refrigerator for up to 3 days.

Asiago

Asiago is a hard cheese usually found near the deli section of your grocery store. It has a distinct taste and is often paired with Parmesan. If Asiago isn't your thing, feel free to top the bagel with Cheddar or your favorite cheese!

QUICK MUG STRAWBERRY SHORTCAKE

Sometimes you don't want to bake a big cake, because portion control can be difficult. This is a single-serving recipe that will satisfy your sweet tooth without leaving you with leftovers to dodge. Low-carb berries can be a nice treat, even on a ketogenic diet. Paired with high-fat whipped cream, this quick dessert will help keep you on track!

Prep time 5 minutes | **Cook time** 2 minutes | **Serves 1**

2 tablespoons unsalted butter

2 tablespoons finely ground blanched almond flour

2 teaspoons coconut flour

3 teaspoons granular erythritol, divided

1 teaspoon vanilla extract

⅛ teaspoon baking powder

1 large egg

¼ cup heavy whipping cream

2 strawberries, sliced

Per Serving
Calories: 526 |
Fat: 49g | Protein: 9g | Sodium: 156mg |
Fiber: 1g | Carbohydrates: 17g |
Sugar Alcohol: 12g |
Net Carbohydrates: 10g | Sugar: 4g

1 In a 10-ounce microwave-safe coffee mug, melt butter in the microwave, about 20 seconds. Add almond flour, coconut flour, and 2 teaspoons erythritol. Whisk in vanilla, baking powder, and egg.

2 Place the mug back into the microwave for 60 seconds. The cake will puff up and feel firm when done. Cook in additional 10-second increments if needed. Let cool for 5 minutes, then run a knife along the sides to remove.

3 In a medium bowl, whisk heavy whipping cream and the remaining teaspoon of erythritol until fluffy whipped cream forms. Cut the cake in half and place half of the whipped cream in between the cake layers along with one sliced strawberry. Place the second half of the cake on top and add the remaining whipped cream and strawberry slices. Serve chilled.

MASON JAR VANILLA ICE CREAM

Ice cream sundaes, anyone? This easy method doesn't require any machinery—only four ingredients and a little bit of elbow grease stand between you and a sweet and creamy dessert!

Prep time 10 minutes | **Cook time** N/A | **Serves 2**

½ cup heavy whipping cream
½ cup unsweetened almond milk
¼ cup powdered erythritol
½ teaspoon vanilla extract

Per Serving
Calories: 215 | Fat: 22g | Protein: 1g | Sodium: 67mg | Fiber: 0g | Carbohydrates: 20g | Sugar Alcohol: 18g | Net Carbohydrates: 11g | Sugar: 2g

1 Place all the ingredients in a 16-ounce Mason jar, put the lid on, and shake until the mixture becomes thick. It'll be done once you can't hear the liquid hitting the lid when you shake it.

2 Place into the freezer for 3 hours, shaking for 30 seconds once every hour. Enjoy with a spoon out of the jar or scoop into two bowls for serving. Serve cold.

Make It Your Own

This recipe makes a great base, but feel free to add your favorite low-carb mix-ins to flavor your ice cream. With fresh strawberries, espresso powder, or even a teaspoon of your favorite extract, the possibilities are endless!

TRIPLE-LAYER CHOCOLATE CAKE

Chocoholics, you have met your match. Perfect for any birthday party, this cake is so moist and decadent that it could even fool your non-keto friends! It's rich enough to be filling but not over-bearingly sweet. The frosting is similar to buttercream in texture, which means it's perfect for getting creative and piping swirls, dots, or your favorite classic cake designs.

Prep time 10 minutes | **Cook time** 20 minutes | **Serves 12**

2 cups finely ground blanched almond flour

½ cup plus 3 tablespoons unsweetened cocoa powder, divided

1 teaspoon baking powder

½ cup salted butter, softened

¾ cup granular erythritol

2 teaspoons vanilla extract, divided

2 large eggs

1 cup unsweetened almond milk

8 ounces cream cheese, softened

½ cup unsalted butter, softened

⅓ cup powdered erythritol

2 tablespoons heavy whipping cream

Per Serving

Calories: 349 | Fat: 32g | Protein: 7g | Sodium: 200mg | Fiber: 4g | Carbohydrates: 27g | Sugar Alcohol: 16g | Net Carbohydrates: 15g | Sugar: 2g

1 Preheat the oven to 350°F.

2 In a large bowl, mix almond flour, ½ cup cocoa powder, and baking powder until fully combined.

3 In a medium bowl, mix salted butter, granular erythritol, and 1 teaspoon vanilla until smooth. Crack open eggs into the bowl and stir until completely combined, then stir in almond milk. Add the wet mixture to the dry ingredients and stir until combined.

4 Prepare three 6" round cake pans (or work in batches if needed). Generously butter or use pan spray to prevent sticking. Then evenly pour batter among three pans.

5 Bake for 20 minutes or until the cakes spring back when you touch them and a toothpick inserted in the centers comes out clean.

6 Let cool completely before removing from the pans or they may fall apart. Allow to cool for a few hours at room temperature, then place in the refrigerator overnight.

7 To make the frosting, whip cream cheese, unsalted butter, powdered erythritol, the remaining vanilla, the remaining cocoa powder, and heavy whipping cream together in a large bowl until fluffy, 3–5 minutes.

8 To assemble, place the first cake on a work surface and spread ⅓ frosting over top. Place second cake layer and add frosting. Repeat with third layer and smooth frosting over top. Slice into twelve pieces and serve chilled.

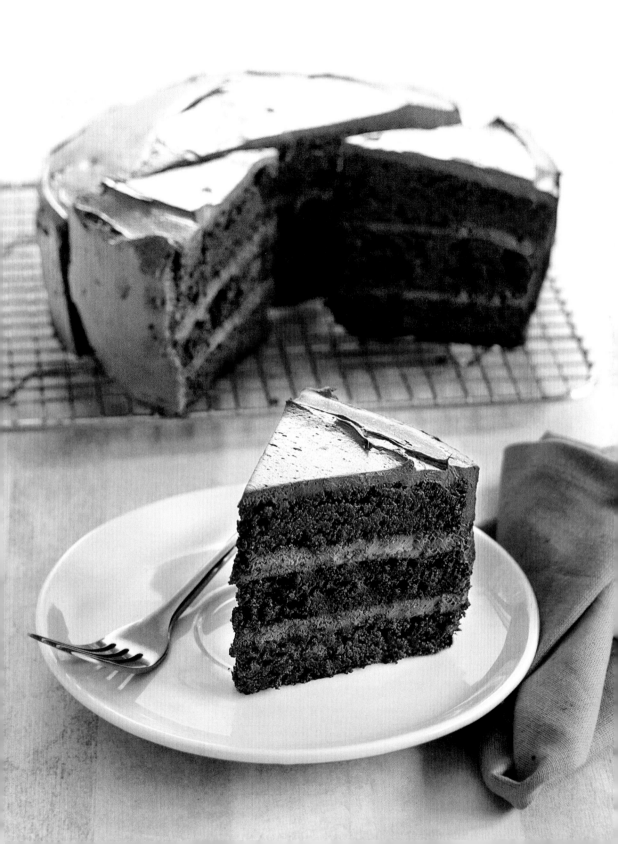

EDIBLE COOKIE DOUGH

Grab a spoon! This recipe contains no egg, so it's totally safe to eat, and with no sugar it's totally keto-friendly. This recipe is great for both kiddos and grown-ups. It has the consistency of traditional cookie dough with slightly more texture from the almond flour. Feel free to add your favorite mix-ins or experiment with different extracts such as caramel or toffee.

Prep time 5 minutes | **Cook time** N/A | **Serves 2**

2 tablespoons powdered erythritol

¼ cup salted butter, softened

½ teaspoon vanilla extract

1 tablespoon no-sugar-added almond butter

½ cup finely ground blanched almond flour

¼ cup low-carb chocolate chips

Per Serving
Calories: 525 | Fat: 49g | Protein: 10g | Sodium: 182mg | Fiber: 12g | Carbohydrates: 34g | Sugar Alcohol: 15g | Net Carbohydrates: 15g | Sugar: 2g

In a medium bowl, beat erythritol, butter, vanilla, and almond butter until fluffy. Add almond flour and beat until combined, about 1 minute. Fold in chocolate chips. Chill for at least 1 hour. Serve chilled.

CHOCOLATE CHIP COOKIES

Desserts don't get much more comforting than a plate of warm chocolate chip cookies. This recipe makes a dozen chewy and delightful cookies that even your non-keto friends (and kids!) will love! Be sure to serve them with a cold glass of almond milk.

Prep time 10 minutes | **Cook time** 15 minutes | **Yields 12, 1 per serving**

4 tablespoons salted butter, melted

½ cup granular erythritol

1 teaspoon vanilla extract

1¼ cups finely ground blanched almond flour

½ teaspoon baking powder

¼ teaspoon baking soda

1 large egg

¼ teaspoon apple cider vinegar

⅓ cup low-carb chocolate chips

Per Serving

Calories: 133 | Fat: 12g | Protein: 4g | Sodium: 82mg | Fiber: 3g | Carbohydrates: 14g | Sugar Alcohol: 9g | Net Carbohydrates: 7g | Sugar: 0g

1 Preheat the oven to 350°F. Line a large baking sheet with parchment paper.

2 In a medium bowl, whisk butter, erythritol, and vanilla, then set aside. In a large bowl, whisk almond flour, baking powder, and baking soda. Add the wet mixture to the dry mixture and use a rubber spatula to mix until combined.

3 Add in egg and mix until combined, then pour in vinegar and fold in chocolate chips.

4 Scoop about 2 tablespoons of the dough and roll into a ball. Place on the prepared baking sheet, and repeat with the remaining dough to make twelve cookies. Press the tops to slightly flatten, then bake for 12 minutes or until edges are golden. Let cool for 20 minutes before moving, otherwise they will fall apart. Serve warm. Store in an air-tight container in the refrigerator up to 4 days.

Avoid Maltitol

Some sugar-free chocolate brands use maltitol or maltitol syrup as the main sweetener. Maltitol is a high-glycemic sweetener that can spike your blood sugar and cause uncomfortable digestive distress. Be sure to check the ingredient label before you buy! Look for chocolate that uses natural sweeteners like stevia. If it's too difficult to find, try buying a 70 or more percent cocoa chocolate bar and breaking it up into chunks.

DOUBLE-CHOCOLATE BROWNIES

These brownies are a chocolate lover's dream! They are rich, fudgy, decadent, and delicious, and they come together in no time at all. Take this recipe to the next level by serving them with a scoop of Mason Jar Vanilla Ice Cream (see recipe in this chapter).

Prep time 10 minutes | **Cook time** 15 minutes | **Serves 12**

½ cup salted butter, softened

½ cup granular erythritol

⅓ cup unsweetened dark cocoa powder

½ teaspoon espresso powder

2 teaspoons vanilla

1¼ cups finely ground blanched almond flour

1 teaspoon baking powder

2 large eggs

½ cup low-carb chocolate chips

Per Serving

Calories: 191 | Fat: 17g | Protein: 5g | Sodium: 113mg | Fiber: 5g | Carbohydrates: 18g | Sugar Alcohol: 10g | Net Carbohydrates: 8g | Sugar: 1g

1 Preheat the oven to 350°F.

2 Place butter, erythritol, cocoa powder, espresso powder, and vanilla in a food processor. Pulse until smooth, about 20 seconds, scraping down the sides as necessary.

3 In a large bowl, mix almond flour and baking powder. Scrape the wet mixture into the dry ingredients, then gently mix until combined. Crack open eggs into a small bowl and whisk, then pour into the batter and stir until combined.

4 Fold chocolate chips into the batter. Pour into a parchment paper–lined 8" × 8" baking dish and bake for 15 minutes or until a toothpick inserted in the center comes out clean. Let cool for at least 1 hour to avoid crumbling. Serve warm. Store in an airtight container in the refrigerator up to 4 days for max freshness.

Cocoa Quality

Using dark unsweetened cocoa powder versus regular will yield significantly different results in the taste of these brownies. Keep that in mind when planning for this recipe. In either case, make sure you're using a fresh pack of cocoa powder to bring out the best chocolaty flavor!

DINNER ROLLS

This recipe delivers the perfect, savory, bread-like side to complement any dish, from a hearty chili (see options in Chapter 3) to Pasta Primavera (see recipe in Chapter 5). Not only is it beyond delicious; it's also incredibly versatile. You can use the rolls as buns for your favorite burger or even bake the dough in a loaf pan to slice for sandwiches. The flax in these rolls could be swapped out for more almond flour, but I highly recommend leaving it in because it truly gives them that wheat roll taste.

Prep time 10 minutes | **Cook time** 15 minutes | **Serves 6**

1 cup shredded mozzarella

2 tablespoons salted butter

1 cup finely ground blanched almond flour

⅓ cup ground golden flax

1 large egg yolk

½ teaspoon baking soda

⅛ teaspoon finely ground pink Himalayan salt

Per Serving
Calories: 262 | Fat: 21g | Protein: 11g | Sodium: 300mg | Fiber: 5g | Carbohydrates: 7g | Net Carbohydrates: 2g | Sugar: 1g

1 Preheat the oven to 400°F. Line a large baking sheet with parchment paper.

2 In a large microwave-safe bowl, mix mozzarella, butter, and almond flour. Microwave for 45 seconds, then stir and microwave for an additional 15 seconds. Stir until a soft ball of dough forms.

3 Mix in flax, egg yolk, baking soda, and salt until well combined. Roll the mixture into a ball, then cut into six even pieces. Roll each piece of dough into a round, flattened disc shape, then place on the prepared baking sheet.

4 Bake for 10–12 minutes or until the edges and tops begin to turn golden. Let cool for 10 minutes before serving. Store in an airtight container in the refrigerator up to 3 days.

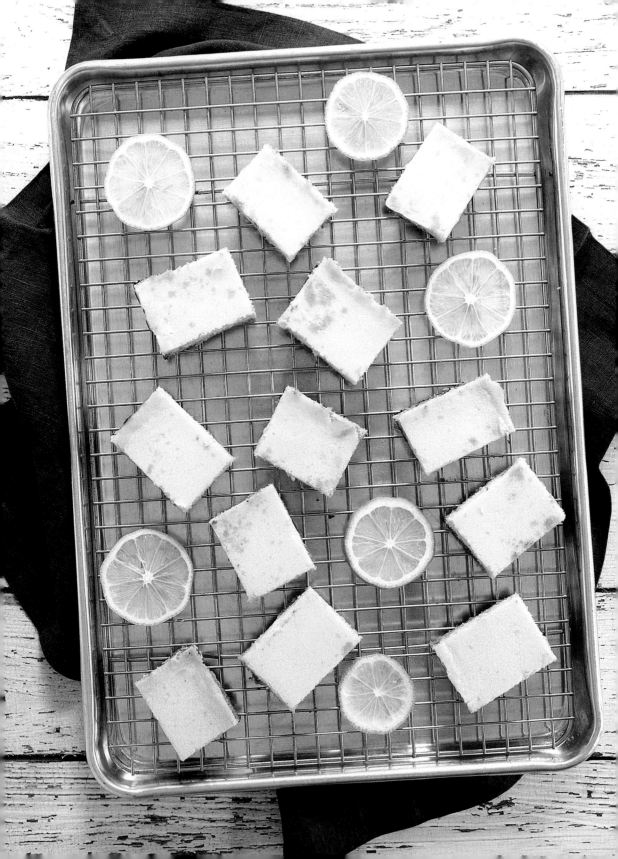

LEMON BARS

This light and tangy dish is the ultimate dessert to break out in the springtime. The buttery crust perfectly complements the tang of the lemon filling, giving you an irresistible sweet treat that you won't want to put down!

Prep time 10 minutes | **Cook time** 25 minutes | **Serves 12**

1½ cups finely ground blanched almond flour

¼ cup salted butter

½ teaspoon vanilla extract

3 large lemons, juiced

3 large eggs

4 ounces cream cheese, softened

½ cup powdered erythritol

2 tablespoons coconut flour

Per Serving
Calories: 176 | Fat: 15g | Protein: 5g | Sodium: 83mg | Fiber: 2g | Carbohydrates: 10g | Sugar Alcohol: 6g | Net Carbohydrates: 5g | Sugar: 1g

1 Preheat the oven to 350°F.

2 In a food processor, pulse almond flour, butter, and vanilla until a crumbly texture similar to sand forms, about ten pulses.

3 Press the mixture into an 8" × 8" baking dish, then bake for 10 minutes or until golden. Let cool completely.

4 In a medium bowl, whisk together lemon juice, eggs, cream cheese, erythritol, and coconut flour. Pour the mixture over the cooled crust, then bake for an additional 15 minutes or until set and lightly browned on the top. Let cool for 1 hour, then cover and chill in the refrigerator for at least 1 hour. Serve chilled.

GARLIC KNOTS

Popular as a side to order with pizza, Garlic Knots are a savory and appetizing treat for your taste buds. Not only is making a bread-free version easier than it might seem; once you're a pro, you can get creative and put your own spin on things! Pair these with a pizza from Chapter 4 for a complete pizza night in.

Prep time 10 minutes | **Cook time** 15 minutes | **Serves 12**

2 cups shredded mozzarella

2 tablespoons unsalted butter

2 cups finely ground blanched almond flour

1½ teaspoons baking powder

1 teaspoon apple cider vinegar

⅛ teaspoon finely ground pink Himalayan salt

2 tablespoons salted butter, melted

3 cloves garlic, peeled and finely minced

1 tablespoon finely chopped fresh parsley

Per Serving
Calories: 205 | Fat: 17g | Protein: 9g | Sodium: 221mg | Fiber: 2g | Carbohydrates: 5g | Net Carbohydrates: 3g | Sugar: 1g

1 Preheat the oven to 400°F. Line a large baking sheet with parchment paper.

2 In a large microwave-safe bowl, mix mozzarella, unsalted butter, and almond flour. Microwave for 45 seconds, then stir. Microwave for an additional 15 seconds, then stir.

3 Mix in baking powder, vinegar, and salt and continue stirring until a soft dough forms. Wet your hands with a bit of water to prevent sticking and knead dough if necessary.

4 Place the ball of dough between two large pieces of parchment paper. Roll into a ½"-thick, 9" × 12" rectangle. Use a pizza cutter to cut into twelve 1"-thick strips.

5 Carefully tie each strip of dough into a knot by looping the ends together, as you would tying a shoelace. Place each knot on the prepared baking sheet.

6 In a small bowl, whisk salted butter and garlic. Gently brush the mixture on each knot and sprinkle with parsley.

7 Bake for 14 minutes or until the knots turn golden. Let them cool for at least 10 minutes. Feel free to serve with your favorite low-carb marinara sauce for dipping.

HAMBURGER BUNS

Bunless burgers are great, but sometimes you just want to enjoy a classic-style burger—bread and all! These Hamburger Buns are filling and quick to bake. They are so delicious that you'll feel like you're enjoying a regular burger but without any of the guilt. You don't need any special pan for this recipe, but if you have a whoopie pie pan, this would be a great recipe to use it on.

Prep time 5 minutes | **Cook time** 15 minutes | **Serves 4**

1½ cups shredded mozzarella

2 ounces cream cheese

1½ cups finely ground blanched almond flour

1 teaspoon baking powder

½ teaspoon apple cider vinegar

1 large egg

2 tablespoons salted butter, melted

2 tablespoons sesame seeds

Per Serving
Calories: 525 | Fat: 43g | Protein: 23g | Sodium: 525mg | Fiber: 5g | Carbohydrates: 12g | Net Carbohydrates: 7g | Sugar: 3g

1 Preheat the oven to 350°F. Line a baking sheet with parchment paper.

2 In a large microwave-safe bowl, add mozzarella, cream cheese, and almond flour. Microwave for 45 seconds, then stir.

3 Microwave for an additional 15 seconds, then add baking powder, vinegar, and egg. Stir until a soft ball of dough forms. Wet your hands to prevent sticking, then separate the dough into four balls.

4 Form into bun shapes by creating a flat disc shape, then place on the prepared baking sheet. They may seem small, but they will increase in size while cooking. Brush each with butter and place sesame seeds on top. Bake for 10–12 minutes or until edges are golden. Let cool for at least 10 minutes before slicing to serve.

SOFT BAKED PRETZELS

Nothing beats a mall pretzel...you know, the soft-baked, bready goodness it seems like you can get only in a food court? Well, this recipe replicates that fluffy dough in a better-for-you version that has a fraction of the carbs. Serve with low-carb cheese sauce, mustard, or marinara sauce.

Prep time 15 minutes | **Cook time** 20 minutes | **Yields 8**

2 cups shredded mozzarella
2 tablespoons unsalted butter
2 cups finely ground blanched almond flour
1½ teaspoons baking powder
1 teaspoon apple cider vinegar
2 tablespoons salted butter
1 large egg, whisked

Per Serving
Calories: 298 | Fat: 24g | Protein: 14g | Sodium: 301mg | Fiber: 3g | Carbohydrates: 7g | Net Carbohydrates: 4g | Sugar: 2g

1 Preheat the oven to 400°F. Line a large baking sheet with parchment paper.

2 In a large microwave-safe bowl, microwave mozzarella and unsalted butter for 1 minute, then stir until melted. Add almond flour and baking powder and stir until a soft ball of dough forms, then stir in vinegar.

3 Separate the dough into two balls, then cut each into four sections. Take one section of the dough and form eight pretzel shapes by twisting the two ends twice, then looping them down to form the classic shape. Repeat with the remaining dough.

4 In a small bowl, whisk salted butter and egg. Brush each pretzel with egg mixture and bake for 15 minutes until dark golden brown. Let cool for 10 minutes. Serve warm.

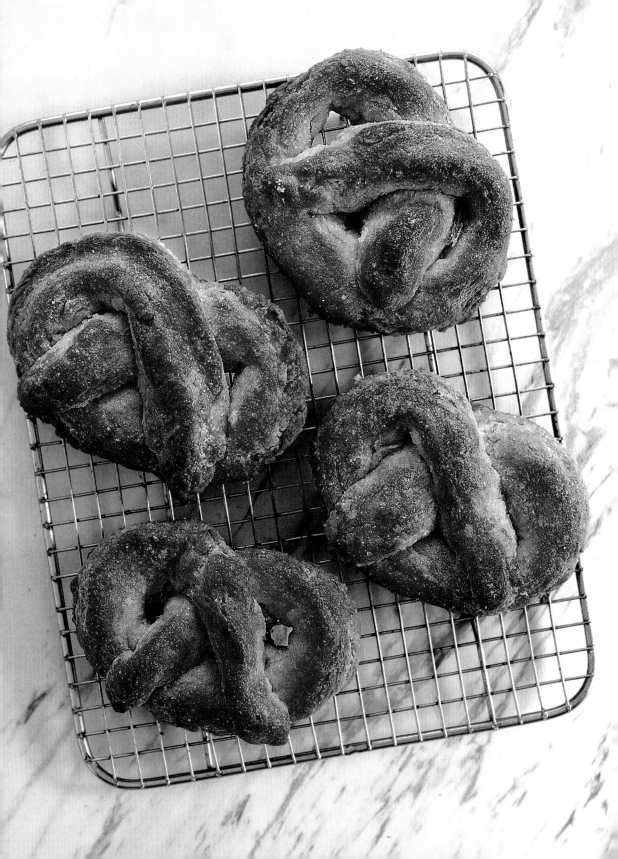

US/METRIC CONVERSION CHART

VOLUME CONVERSIONS

US Volume Measure	Metric Equivalent
⅛ teaspoon	0.5 milliliter
¼ teaspoon	1 milliliter
½ teaspoon	2 milliliters
1 teaspoon	5 milliliters
½ tablespoon	7 milliliters
1 tablespoon (3 teaspoons)	15 milliliters
2 tablespoons (1 fluid ounce)	30 milliliters
¼ cup (4 tablespoons)	60 milliliters
⅓ cup	90 milliliters
½ cup (4 fluid ounces)	125 milliliters
⅔ cup	160 milliliters
¾ cup (6 fluid ounces)	180 milliliters
1 cup (16 tablespoons)	250 milliliters
1 pint (2 cups)	500 milliliters
1 quart (4 cups)	1 liter (about)

WEIGHT CONVERSIONS

US Weight Measure	Metric Equivalent
½ ounce	15 grams
1 ounce	30 grams
2 ounces	60 grams
3 ounces	85 grams
¼ pound (4 ounces)	115 grams
½ pound (8 ounces)	225 grams
¾ pound (12 ounces)	340 grams
1 pound (16 ounces)	454 grams

OVEN TEMPERATURE CONVERSIONS

Degrees Fahrenheit	Degrees Celsius
200 degrees F	95 degrees C
250 degrees F	120 degrees C
275 degrees F	135 degrees C
300 degrees F	150 degrees C
325 degrees F	160 degrees C
350 degrees F	180 degrees C
375 degrees F	190 degrees C
400 degrees F	205 degrees C
425 degrees F	220 degrees C
450 degrees F	230 degrees C

BAKING PAN SIZES

American	Metric
8 x 1½ inch round baking pan	20 x 4 cm cake tin
9 x 1½ inch round baking pan	23 x 3.5 cm cake tin
11 x 7 x 1½ inch baking pan	28 x 18 x 4 cm baking tin
13 x 9 x 2 inch baking pan	30 x 20 x 5 cm baking tin
2 quart rectangular baking dish	30 x 20 x 3 cm baking tin
15 x 10 x 2 inch baking pan	30 x 25 x 2 cm baking tin (Swiss roll tin)
9 inch pie plate	22 x 4 or 23 x 4 cm pie plate
7 or 8 inch springform pan	18 or 20 cm springform or loose bottom cake tin
9 x 5 x 3 inch loaf pan	23 x 13 x 7 cm or 2 lb narrow loaf or paté tin
1½ quart casserole	1.5 liter casserole
2 quart casserole	2 liter casserole

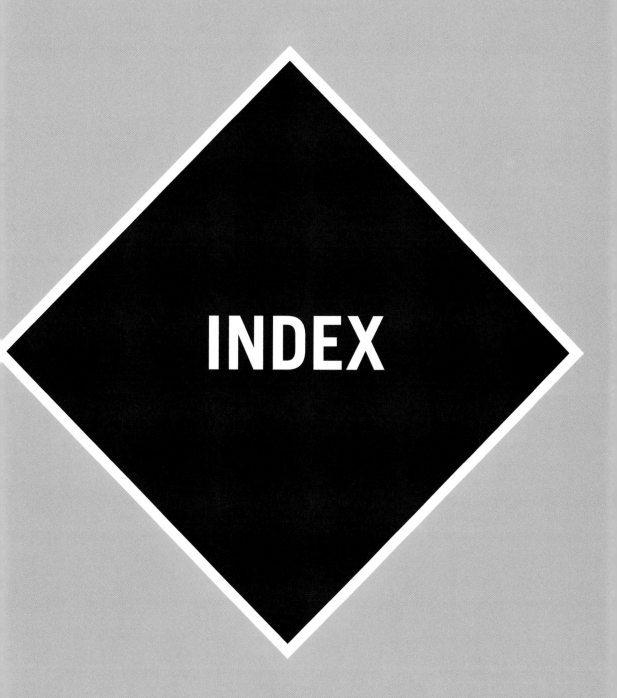

INDEX

Stick to your keto diet WITHOUT giving up your favorite foods!

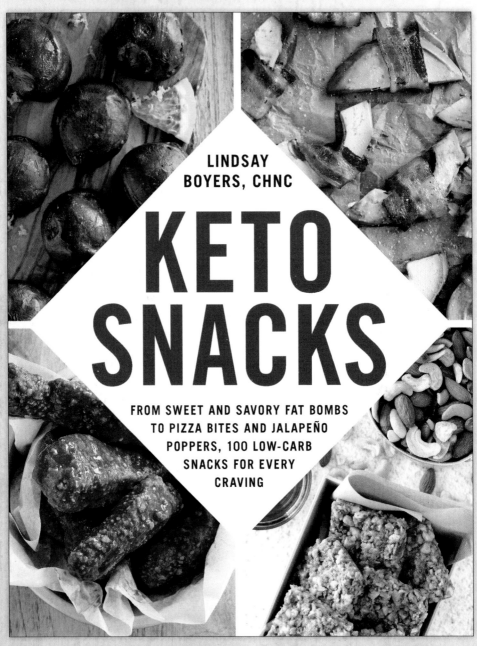

LINDSAY
BOYERS, CHNC

KETO SNACKS

FROM SWEET AND SAVORY FAT BOMBS
TO PIZZA BITES AND JALAPEÑO
POPPERS, 100 LOW-CARB
SNACKS FOR EVERY
CRAVING

Pick up or download your copy today!

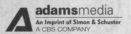

adamsmedia
An Imprint of Simon & Schuster
A CBS COMPANY